Contents

List of Figures v

Introduction vi

1. Approaching the problem of voices 1

    1.1 A few words about meaning 4

    1.2 Understanding voices: the overall picture 6

2. For voice-hearers **21**

    2.1 About voices 23

    2.2 Things that give your voice power 25

    2.3 The first step: changing the way that you think about voices 30

    2.4 The second step: getting to know your voices 34

    2.5 The third step: paying attention to your self-worth 36

    2.6 Special tricks 40

    2.7 Summary of voice-hearers section 46

3. For clinicians **49**

    3.1 What should I do? 53

    3.2 Your orientation and attitude 57

    3.3 Practical stuff 62

4. For carers and family **83**

    4.1 Loss 85

    4.2 What you will be facing 88

    4.3 The relationship has changed – what should I do? 93

    4.4 What should I do about engaging? 94

    4.5 What should I do with my voice-hearer's voices? 98

5. In conclusion **107**

    5.1 Guidance notes taken from chapters 110

Appendices **117**

Appendix 1: Self-worth 119

Appendix 2: Assertiveness..120

Appendix 3: Strategic overview..121

Appendix 4: Emergencies flowchart 122

Appendix 5: Patsy Hage's story 123

Appendix 6: My history of hearing voices 124

Appendix 7: Voices rap sheet 126

Appendix 8: Strategies that you use to deal with your voices 128

Appendix 9: Getting my life back..129

Appendix 10: Relapse prevention 130

References 131

Index..137

> *There are no facts, only interpretations.*
>
> Friedrich Nietzsche
>
> *When I loved myself enough*
> *I stopped trying to banish the critical voices from my head.*
> *Now I say, 'Thank you for your views'*
> *and they feel heard ...*
> *End of discussion.*
>
> Kim McMillen

List of figures

Figure 1   Personal interpretations and meanings 5

Figure 2   Relationships linked to voice-hearer 9

Figure 3   Spectrum of feelings 13

Figure 4   Feelings – thoughts – actions cycle 14

Figure 5   The effect of repeated avoidance on anxiety, adapted
           from Powell (1992) 18

Figure 6   Power slots in a relationship 73

Introduction

In the interests of keeping this book uncomplicated, when I speak of 'voices' I generally mean troublesome voices, which should be distinguished from voices that are not troublesome to the person hearing them.

The book is split into three core sections, each speaking to a different audience, because — although different — the approaches used by these three audiences should best work together. Each section is tailored to fit those particular readers' understanding of the subject, and there has necessarily been some overlap.

People have been hearing voices through the ages. Some people have difficulty with these experiences; other people do not. It is not the hearing of voices that causes difficulties; it is how the person having these experiences responds to them. Thus, it is the type of response that, in turn, will define the experience as troublesome or not. This is true of any relationship.

It is important to know that voices can occur in the following instances and are considered normal:

- when deprived of sleep for several days
- when suffering from certain physical illness conditions, such as a prolonged fever
- when suffering from certain organic disorders
- within a particular cultural context; for example, Native North Americans and the Zulu sangoma (Southern African traditional healers) who have contact with ancestors.

There are also people who hear voices but who can get on with their lives. I will go into this phenomenon later. However, what I would like to stress is that it is often difficult to distinguish between 'normal' and 'not normal'. That is, why so few have ventured to define 'normality'. Maslow and Mittelmann (1951) made an attempt at this that I think is a good starting point. They defined normality along the lines of the following, which I have adapted to be more understandable:

- It is important that I feel more or less OK about myself.
- I should have some picture of and awareness about myself.
- I should have life goals and these should be realistic.
- I need to have a realistic and practical view of the social system in which I live.

- My personality should be more or less constant and predictable.
- My experiences should help me deal with life.
- I should be able to act naturally without losing focus.
- I should be able to express feelings in a rational way.
- I need to be able to participate in group activities, but not at the expense of my individuality.
- I need to have awareness of my physical needs, which I should satisfy within the norms of society.

Troublesome voices cause disruption in almost every one of these areas.

It is interesting to speculate that Maslow and Mittelmann perhaps did not realise that what they were describing would most likely today be called resilience factors[1]. It is also interesting to note that these factors could be seen as goals in life.

To this end, the Buckinghamshire Early Intervention Service (BEIS), in which I was the clinical lead, developed a statement of recovery (2007a, p13). Recovery is viewed as:

- functioning independently: having definite and achievable goals and actively pursuing them with minimum support from mental health services
- having constructive control over symptoms so that there is little or no disabling effect present
- constructive control, as described above, being present without interruption for at least six months.

As mentioned, in this book I focus on troublesome voices. The aim of the book is to introduce voice-hearers and their carers and clinicians with whom they may be involved to ways of dealing with troublesome voices.

Those who are troubled by their voices have limited and, for the most part, ineffective strategies for dealing with their voices. While trying to deal with them they are so trampled by their voices that they do not even know where to start applying those few strategies that they have in a coherent way.

The carers of people troubled by voices are like people who have been savaged by a heavyweight boxer and for most of the time are reeling under the impact. They, too, have no effective guidance and, try as hard as they may, often do the incorrect thing, thereby upsetting the situation further.

Surprisingly, barring a few experts, clinicians in the field are in a similar boat to carers. Clinicians are often the people at the pit face and as such are expected to be people who 'should know'. However, certainly over of all my time working in acute mental health, most clinicians suffered as much through lack of practical and effective techniques.

The approaches I will be discussing can be used whenever voices arrive, by voice-hearers, carers and clinicians alike. Each of these groups will, however, approach the problem from a slightly different perspective. These approaches should help the person and those around them to regain control of their lives.

The book thus presents a three-pronged attack on voices. If all of these elements are available, it is of the utmost importance that voice-hearers, carers and clinicians work together as a system. However, at the end of the day, it is the voice-hearer who will make the most dynamic impact on overcoming troublesome voices.

Material for the book was extensively derived directly from my work with voice-hearers over the last decade of my working life in an acute mental health setting as well as being clinical lead in the Buckinghamshire Early Intervention Service. I do, however, draw on what I consider to be seminal approaches to dealing with voices and helping voice-hearers. Chiefly, these are cognitive, cognitive behavioural, client-centred, group and interpersonal therapy, as well as the mindfulness and compassionate mind approaches.

On the Frontline with Voices

A grassroots handbook for voice-hearers, carers and clinicians

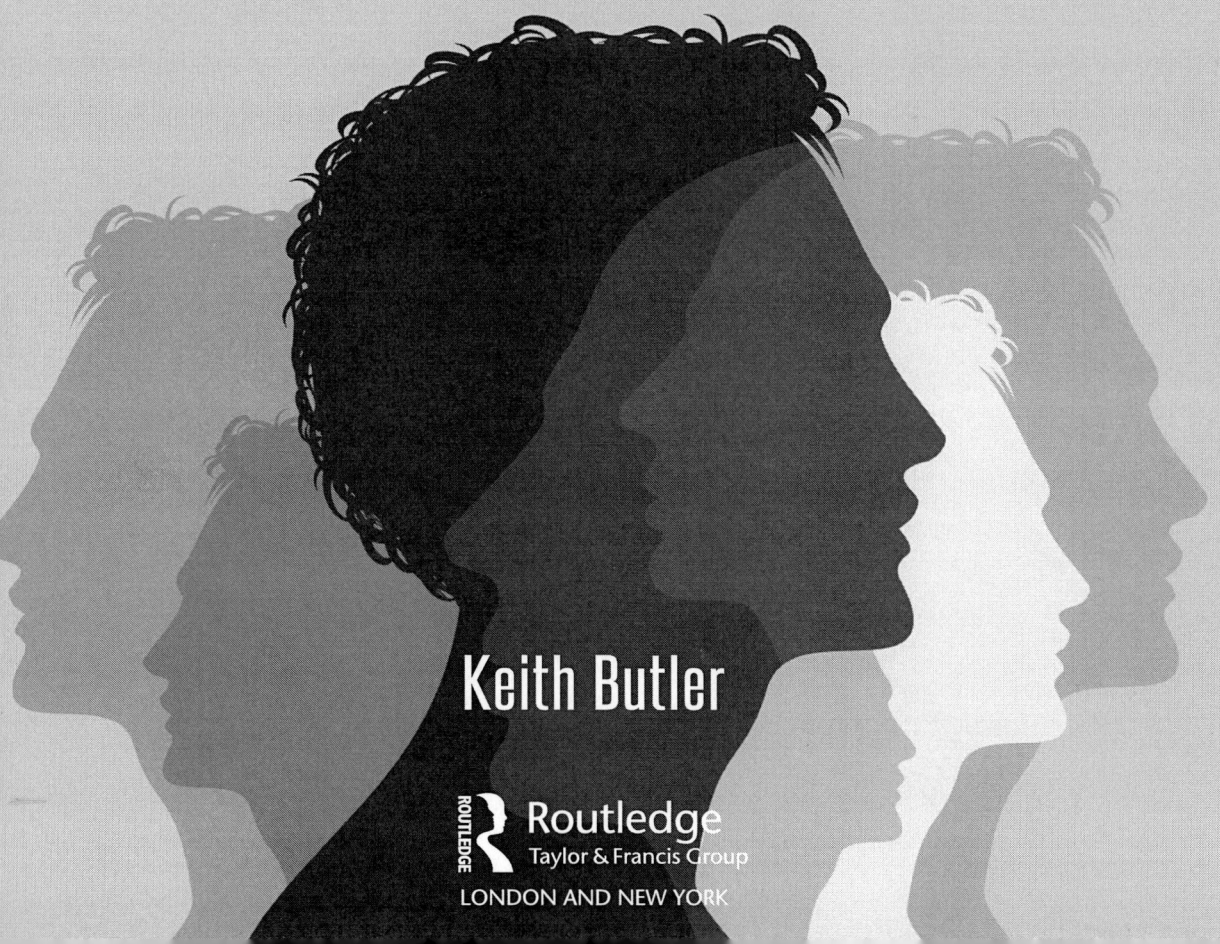

Keith Butler

Routledge
Taylor & Francis Group

LONDON AND NEW YORK

Dedication

To Lynette and Jessica … for walking the road with me.

First published 2016 by Speechmark Publishing Ltd.

Published 2017 by Routledge
2 Park Square, Milton Park, Abingdon, Oxon OX14 4RN
711 Third Avenue, New York, NY 10017, USA

Routledge is an imprint of the Taylor & Francis Group, an informa business

Design and artwork by Moo Creative (Luton)

British Library Cataloguing in Publication Data
A catalogue record for this book is available from the British Library

ISBN 9781909301696 (pbk)

Chapter 1

Approaching the problem of voices

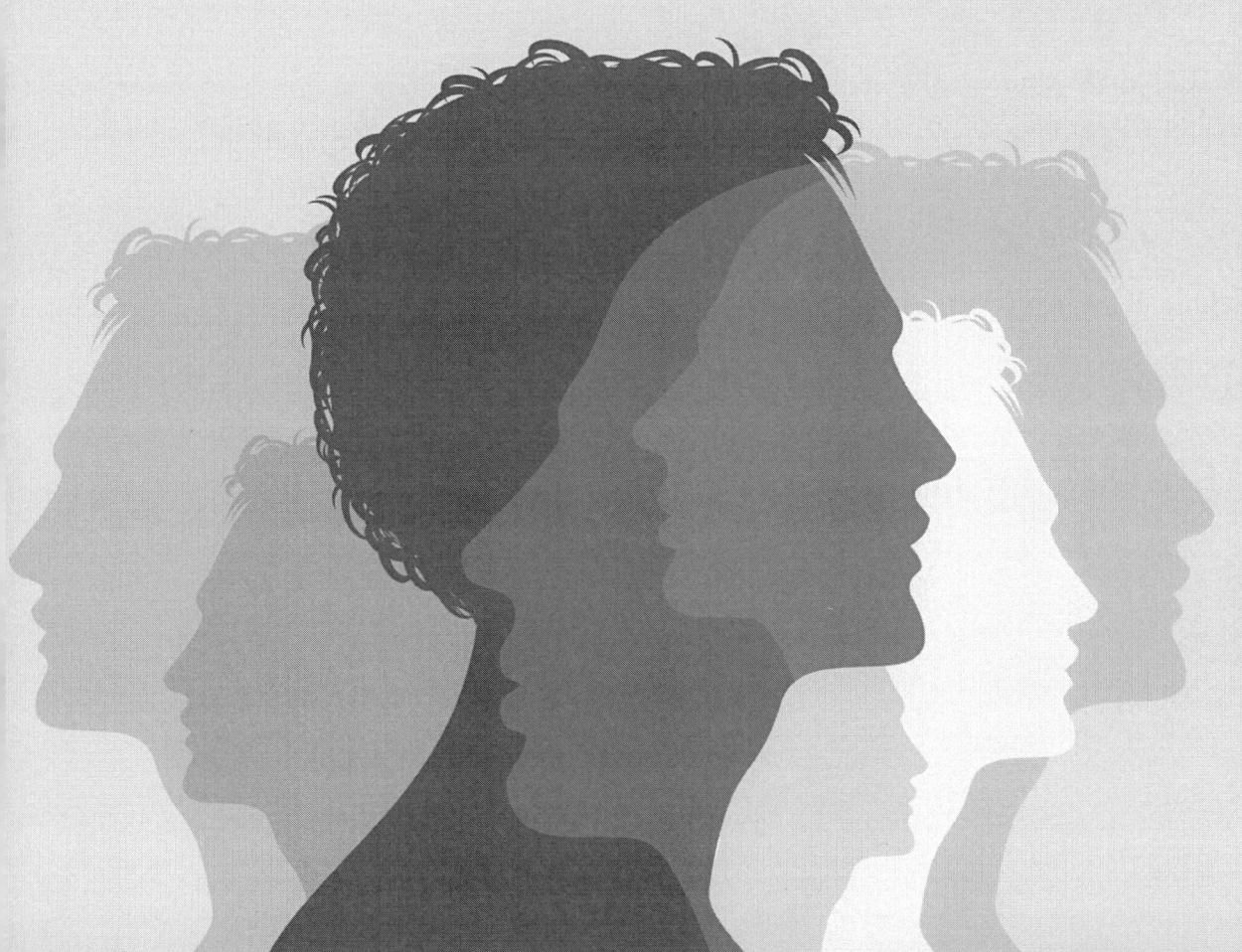

Approaching the problem of voices

The Western view of hearing voices – commonly referred to as auditory hallucinations in the mental health world – has for many years been embedded in psychiatry. In other words, descriptions of cause were only presented as biological. Consequently, the chief recommendation for treatment has until recently been biological. Medication is given to a patient without the patient really understanding how it works, and therefore being unable to regulate or participate as an equal in the treatment process.

Generally, although the causes are recognised as being complex, models used have presented a somewhat linear picture of cause, effect and treatment. This may be adequate for many medical problems but in matters relating to how people are dealing with thoughts and feelings and the behavioural outcome within the complexities of society there needs to be more thinking in terms of systems. Key issues relating to, for example, the influence of challenging social pressures in the genesis and maintenance of the problem have not been factored into the description. Consequently, the need to intervene in these areas has been underplayed.

Thus, we can say that finding the cause of complex mental health issues is not simple because it is usually multifaceted.

Susan Jeffers (1991) has a noteworthy approach to the problem of cause:

> *But does it really matter where our self doubts come from? I believe not. It is not my approach to analyze the whys and wherefores of troublesome areas of the mind. It is often impossible to figure out what the actual causes of negative patterns are, and even if we did know, the knowing does not necessarily change them. I believe that if something is troubling you, simply start from where you are and take the necessary action to change it.*
> (Jeffers, 1991, 18)

Among others, it is this multifaceted quality of the problem of cause that draws in a psycho-social approach [2]. Decades of crusading to get recognition of psycho-social explanations has eventually born fruit. This innovation has made it easier to describe voice-hearing to people who hear troublesome voices in an understandable way and also to provide them with the tools that

R Routledge
Taylor & Francis Group

they can use on a daily, hourly or even minute-by-minute basis to deal with their voices. In this way, control and power is placed back into their hands.

I therefore want to introduce you to a way of seeing voices that has helped many people move towards an ordinary life where voices may still be present but have become minimally or no longer troublesome to them.

I will be drawing on some key approaches and also strategies that my voice-hearing clients have taught me in individual, group and family therapy settings.

> **The key target is the inherent power dynamic that plays out chiefly within the relationship the voice-hearer has with their voices.**

To make a beginning, I would like you to start thinking like a commander in the army. Before action is taken, a good commander will gather intelligence about the enemy by trying to understand them. At first, this will be an overall picture, and later the commander will try to understand the specifics of the enemy, such as how they fight and what their strong points and weak points are. Having this information at hand allows the astute commander to draw on a variety of techniques and strategies to counteract attack or intrusion.

It is similarly important for people who have to deal with troublesome voices – the voice-hearer, the carer and the clinicians – to adopt a strategic attitude in attempting to overcome voices. They will soon also realise that they will be entering the world of interpretations and meanings that are attached to the experience. This then is perhaps a good place to start.

1.1 A few words about meaning

The various meanings that we place on all our experiences are reflected in the descriptions we attach to them. Some people may say that a ride on a roller coaster is fantastic; others may say that it was horrible. It is the same roller coaster but experienced differently by different people. Thus, it has different meanings to different people and so people respond to it in different ways.

It is quite usual that the meanings each of us attaches to experiences may stay with us for many years, if not our whole lives. For instance, when you hear the word 'apple', what sort of things come into your mind? The sort of things that come into my mind are: eat, bake, sweet, sour, hard, throw, rotten, worms, red, green, skin, bitter, tree, my first apple, primary school, teacher and Snow White. Memories associated with these particular words come to the surface.

 Ɽ Routledge
Taylor & Francis Group

Thus, around almost every word we know or experience we have had there is a halo of personal interpretations, meanings, memories and associations that influence how we see the object – in this case 'apple' (see Figure 1). This then colours the way we behave towards the object – in this case, what we have named 'apple'.

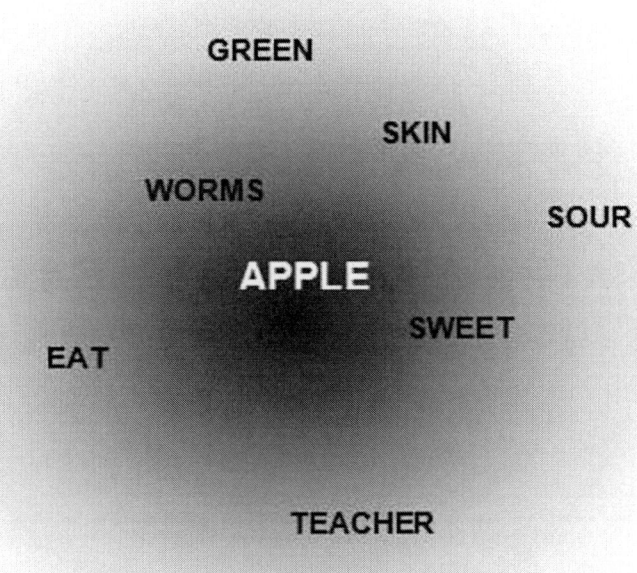

Figure 1 Personal interpretations and meanings

As you can see, there are a lot of memories and experiences locked up for me in this single word 'apple', and so it is for everyone. In other words, if I was blindfolded and given something to taste and it tasted somewhat sour but also had some sweetness, had a bit of a tough bitter skin and a particular smell, I would probably identify it as 'apple'.

What about words like 'father', 'family' or 'dog'? What memories and meanings would then come up for each of us? The only thing we can really say is that they would probably be quite different for each of us.

In each concept, for example, father, dog and even apple, we would have some good memories and meanings and some bad memories and meanings. Whatever the case, every time I see or

Routledge
Taylor & Francis Group

hear someone who, for instance, reminds me of my father, it is quite likely that some of the meanings I attached to that person would come up.

Thus, when any one of us experiences something, one of the first steps our mind takes is to try to make sense of that thing – the 'What is it?', 'Where does it come from?' and so on set of questions pops up. If we cannot immediately make sense of it, our minds still have to try to answer these questions anyway, simply because we do not easily live in a world that is full of questions and strange, unknown experiences. Further, if you do not know what you are experiencing, it is very difficult to know how to respond to it.

So, if I do not know what it is that I am seeing or hearing, I will probably classify it as something closest to what I already know – like the saying: 'If it looks like a duck, sounds like a duck, and walks like a duck, it probably is a duck.' What follows then is that I would interact with this thing as if it is a duck. But with voices it is not that simple. One of my clients illustrated this by reporting that his one voice sounded like his father, but that his father would never say those kinds of things to him.

> **The meanings that voice-hearers attach to their voices play a big role in the way they experience them and thus in the way that they deal with them.**

1.2 Understanding voices: the overall picture

There are many ways to try to understand what voices are so that they can be dealt with in a way that has the least impact on the person's life. As mentioned, the traditional way derives from a medical approach in which voices are described as having biological roots. The most common explanation I have come across is that they are part of a brain disease, in which there is a 'chemical imbalance in the brain'. In order to address this view, the hearing of voices is classified as being part of an illness. Consequently, people become medical patients and are given medication as the first-line treatment.

For me as a psychologist, it does not matter what voices 'really' are. In other words, questions like 'Are voices just caused by a bunch of chemicals or is there some part of the brain that needs to be treated in some way?' are largely irrelevant because there are few current treatments in those domains that offer a life similar to the one had before the person heard voices. What matters in the long run is having a way of dealing with them so that the person can get on with the business of living as soon as possible.

R Routledge
Taylor & Francis Group

There is another very important issue that has to do with what voices are. The dividing line between voices in the clinical sense and other voice-like experiences is very thin. There are some who will no doubt be able to stick a glossy label on what I am about to describe, however this personal experience is hugely troublesome and it affects my behaviour at times. The clever label I have heard it called is 'imposterism'.

Some say that it is more common in girls, but there is a percentage of guys that experience it as well.

My imposterism goes something like this. I do not experience a voice as such but, at the lowest end of the scale, I experience a groundless sense of guilt and culpability when I see a police car. At the rough end of the spectrum with certain experiences, I have intense self-condemning thoughts that may be triggered by the situation or that may arise completely out of the blue. They confront me like a prosecuting barrister with a string of accusations of misrepresenting facts as well as myself, hence the word 'imposterism'. There is a strong feeling that my guilty secret will be discovered and that there will be severe consequences. I have no guilty secret that I know of. However, once on a roll this process is relentless. It can actually cause me to start talking in a defensive way. I almost messed up an important job interview when this process kicked off during the interview. But these are not voices, simply because *I do not actually hear a voice*; they are thoughts and fear responses and I can fairly easily work out what life events are triggering them.

For the voice-hearer, on the other hand, voices are the worst kind of nightmare. They are experienced just as real as when two people are talking to each other. For the voice-hearer the personal origin of their voices is obscure and, as such, an explanation is not readily available. Being thus shrouded in mystery also grants the voice power. Later, you will see that this cloak of mystery is also one of the targets that can be fruitfully attacked.

They subjugate the voice-hearer to a bombardment of criticism, threats and abuse, the likes of which those who have never experienced hearing a voice(s) can barely understand. I could only get an impression of it after many years of work with voice-hearers.

Voices often come at unexpected times, causing the person to feel startled (see section 1.2). They will find themselves waiting for their voices, even when they start learning how to deal with them. After hearing voices constantly for more than 20 years, one voice-hearer described the cessation of voice-hearing as if 'part of his brain was missing'.

Routledge
Taylor & Francis Group

When voices arrive, either as if coming from a distance or by gatecrashing a voice-hearer's thoughts, one by one or all together, the interruption is instant and total. The effect is a bloodless coup in which the person may become instantly and totally overwhelmed. I have seen a client move from productive involvement in a group to being reduced to a sweating, helpless person literally within a minute, for no reason apparent to anyone else in the group. He asked to be left alone for a while and the group continued. Several minutes later he emerged from his battle saying that he had applied the strategies that he had learned and with great effort and tenacity he had reduced his voices to a bearable level. In those few minutes he had overcome his voices.

The person who hears voices easily becomes extremely fearful of them. Often they may feel that they have to obey them and that the voices may never be challenged.

A person who hears voices often believes that their voices are all powerful.

Sometimes it seems that some voice-hearers make a sort of devil's pact with their voices, believing that if they do what the voices ask, they will be left alone. Of course, the anticipated result does not happen. Further, although the voices break this silent contract repeatedly, the voice-hearer may well still believe that it will work sometime. It never does.

One very important issue about voices and emotions is that voices seem to thrive when emotions are aroused. It is for this reason that the group of major tranquilliser drugs are used in the biological management of symptoms. I am grateful that they are available, but these chemicals have to be taken for an extended period and they are not without side effects. The psychological approach to dealing with emotions is to self-limit arousal. Many forms of therapy and counselling train people to do this. Probably the most difficult emotion to deal with is anxiety.

When a voice-hearer becomes anxious, it is highly likely that their voices will be triggered. If the voices are already present, they will most likely get a lot worse. One may then think that voice-hearers could use this aspect to manipulate those around them to never say or do anything that may upset them. However, this is commonly not the case with voice-hearers. The effect of voices dropping in on a voice-hearer is so immediate as to totally limit any cunning the person may have. There is no manipulation. There is no guile. People who pretend to hear voices in order to get some or other gain usually give a very poor performance.

Routledge
Taylor & Francis Group

When tackling voices it is helpful to be aware of how various relationships are linked because the target in voice-hearing is the power relationship between the voice-hearer and the voices. This can be very productively tackled from three areas: the voice-hearer, the carers and the clinicians who may be involved – or, seen another way, whoever is available to aid the voice-hearer. But there is a condition attached, which a diagram (see Figure 2) will explain.

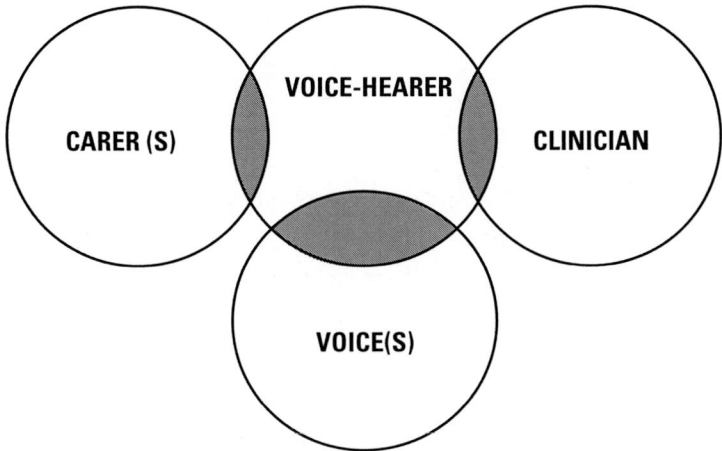

Figure 2 Relationships linked to voice-hearer

Notes

1   The overlapping grey areas indicate points where there are relationships. It illustrates that it is only the voice-hearer who has a relationship with the voice. This highlights the key role of this relationship and that all contributions to the situation by voices, carers or clinicians will go via the voice-hearer.

2   The target of the approach is the type of relationship that the voice-hearer has with the voice. This is no different from helping any person with any troublesome relationship in which the main feature is power and domination. In particular it addresses the question: Who makes the choices about the voice-hearer's behaviour – the voice-hearer or the voice?

The techniques I used focused on:

* the way that the voice-hearer thinks and feels about an experience, including the meaning that they attach to the voice-hearing experience

* the way that the voice-hearer deals with or reacts to this experience

* becoming aware of which of these reactions don't work and changing them into responses that work better, or not using them at all. (Note: a reaction is knee-jerk whereas a response has forethought.)

Routledge Taylor & Francis Group

I remember a person I met at a conference on voice-hearing in London saying that she had not heard her voices for a number of years. I remarked that it seemed as if the voices had gone. Wisely she added, 'I don't want to believe that; but just in case they come back, I have a load of tricks I can play on them.' That was one of the most refreshing statements I have ever heard and it encouraged me to continue working in this difficult field.

It was also at this conference that I first came across the work of Professor Marius Romme and Sandra Escher.

Romme's (1998) research findings highlighted that there are ways in which voices can be dealt with in order to limit their effect on voice-hearers. He discovered and developed these strategies while working with one of his clients, Patsy Hage, in the Netherlands. Patsy heard voices that commanded her to harm herself. Nothing Professor Romme did seemed to help her.

After some time he noticed that she was improving but he could find no explanation for it. Eventually, he discussed this with her and she revealed that she had developed certain ways of responding to her voices and that these ways were making a difference to her life (see Appendix 5: Patsy Hage's story).

To cut a long story short, Professor Romme and Patsy eventually appeared on a TV show in the Netherlands. There was an overwhelming response and this led Professor Romme to realise that there seemed to be two groups of voice-hearers: those who heard voices and did not cope and those who heard voices and did cope (see Table 1). He resolved to discover what caused these differences and conducted research with several hundred volunteers.

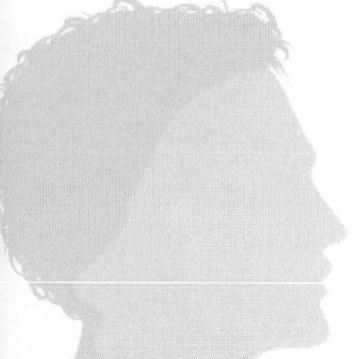

Routledge Taylor & Francis Group

Table 1: Romme's findings (1998): Differences between those who cope and those who do not cope with voice-hearing

People who *do not* cope	People who *do* cope
These people believe that the voices are more powerful than what they actually are.	These people have proved, and therefore know, that the voices are not that powerful.
These people see their voices only as negative and seldom recognise the presence of 'positive' voices.	These people can see their voices in a different light. They are able to recognise 'positive' voices.
These people experience what their voices say as commands.	These people experience what their voices say more as statements or opinions and seldom as commands.
These people never challenge their voices or, alternatively, attack their voices with abuse.	These people attempt to conduct an assertive conversation with their voices and set limits as to the influence the voices have in the relationship.
These people isolate themselves with their voices.	These people communicate fairly often about their voices.
These people chiefly use distraction or avoidance as a psychological strategy.	These people commonly use focusing (non-avoidance) strategies.

Source: Romme, 1998.

Because of the way that they have learned to deal with their voices, people who cope with them have developed the following beliefs:

- The voices are not more powerful than what they are. (Once they have learned this, they respond differently towards their voices.)
- The voices do not always have to be seen as negative. (n other words, they have changed the way that they see them; they have attached a different meaning to them.)
- They are able and, in a sense, allowed, to challenge their voices.
- They can stop isolating themselves with their voices and are prepared to talk to others about them.

Routledge
Taylor & Francis Group

The voice-hearers who coped have, in effect, changed their relationship with their voices on many levels. They are no longer one-down, unassertive and submissive. They have become equal, making choices about their lives, and challenging many of the things that voices say.

Another finding by Romme (1998) of great significance was that there are three stages in the experience of hearing voices:

- **Stage 1: startling phase:** the first time that a person becomes aware of hearing voices is a moment they will seldom forget. It is frightening and causes huge anxiety. They are shockingly startled, hence the name of this phase. It is not unusual that the person remains trapped in this phase for a long period of time – even for their entire lives. Consequently, every time they hear their voices, they experience some of the same frightening emotions.
- **Stage 2: the phase of organisation:** coping with the voices: the person is starting to apply a variety of strategies. Many of the strategies that they apply initially – such as expressing anger or trying to ignore the voices in a variety of ways – either do not work at all or only work for a short period.
- **Stage 3: phase of stabilisation:** the person has integrated their voices as being part of their experience. Their voices are a part of their life, and some of the voices can even be seen to be a positive influence. For example, one person could see her voices as pointing out (through their critical remarks) places in her life that she could improve on, if she wished. In this phase the person is able to exercise a choice about following the advice (instructions) of their voices, or following their own preferences. They no longer slavishly follow their voices; they are in control of their own behaviour.

Romme's findings are extremely important because they suggest the existence of practical strategies that can set the stage for the voice-hearer to take up a life again.

Apart from examining Romme's indispensable findings, my training also focused on what we do with our emotions, the way that we think about things and how we act on our thoughts and emotions. It would help if you had some basic understanding of this. So before I discuss voices, perhaps it is best to say a little bit about feelings (emotions), thoughts and actions (behaviour).

Emotions, thoughts and actions

Emotions are feelings, for example, anger, fear, frustration, happiness, sadness and depression. Thoughts are your conscious reasoning – what you think about. Actions are purely what you do; actions may be planned or spontaneous. Emotions, thoughts and actions are linked to one

Routledge
Taylor & Francis Group

another like a circle of dominoes: should one fall, it could disrupt the stability of at least some of the others. I have described how this works to my clients as follows:

- There are only three basic emotional states; I either feel not-OK, OK or in a state that is somewhere between these two.
- When something affects me it does so by causing a shift between these three emotional states.
- When I feel not-OK, a need arises to change that feeling. The change should take me closer to feeling OK. A common description in psychology is that of needing to reduce tension.
- The smart bit of the kit in my head does not seem to be entirely satisfied with this simple description because it may suggest that a person moves straight from a feeling to an action. This is not the case. Somewhere between emotions and actions we have questions like: 'What exactly am I feeling?' and 'What made me feel not-OK?' and 'How should I deal with the feeling and the situation?' This all happens very quickly and we are largely unaware of the process.
- The 'How should I deal with the feeling and the situation?' question can take one of two directions: I can either stick the whole experience back into my head and think about it a bit longer or I can act on it.
- The action (behaviour) that comes out of this has one chief aim: to reduce the tension. In other words, the not-OK feeling must be reduced. However, it has to do so in such a way that other not-OK feelings are not produced in the process. If this happens, the whole balance will once again be thrown out. Thus, in run-of-the-mill, everyday situations the action has to be a reasonable, social response.

This circular path as described is the ideal. Unfortunately, nothing is perfect. Because there are (at least) several steps in this pathway, they provide places where interference can creep in. Voices do exactly that. It may even be accurate to say that they can interfere at almost every stage of this process. Thus, it could be useful to have a look at this process again, because if we can pin down where a fault is occurring, we are closer to neutralising the fault, or at least limiting its effect. A drawing will help to understand this (see Figure 3).

This is the picture I use to understand the spectrum of feelings:

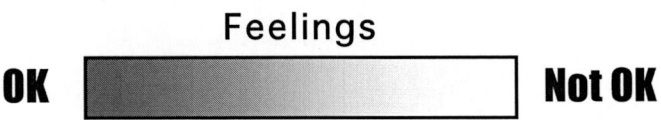

Figure 3 Spectrum of feelings

My feelings can range anywhere along this spectrum. When an event happens, this is how I think about the process. Many of my clients liked this model and used it often to make changes in the way that they deal with life's problems (see Figure 4).

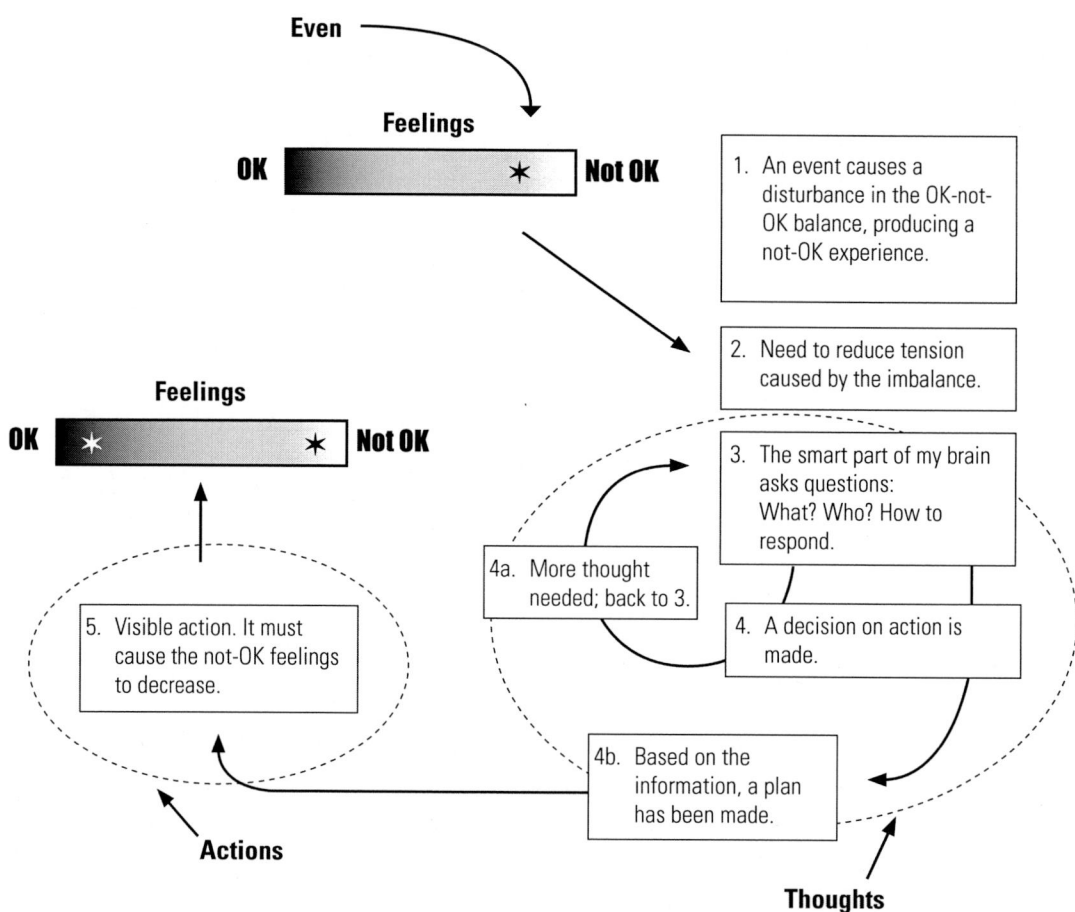

Figure 4   Feelings – thoughts – actions cycle

You will see that in these several steps there are a number of things that can clog up the system. To me, the one that is a prime candidate is at point 4a. Here the process of recycling the thought can go on for a long time and result in no effective action. If, for instance, I keep on believing that the solution I am trying to create will not work and I discard or devalue all solutions that I think of, I then get stuck in my own thoughts. Perhaps a pertinent example of which would be that if I keep reviewing my failures in dealing with my voices, I can come to believe that my voices can never be tamed.

Things can also go wrong at step 5 (the visible action phase). If the action you produce actually causes more distress than the level you were originally experiencing then life just becomes more miserable. There are many voice-hearers who self-harm and/or abuse substances as a way of trying to deal with voices. Clearly these strategies do little or nothing to deal with voices in the longer term and they are also potentially dangerous and personally disrespectful.

There are also some less obvious points in the feelings–thoughts–actions cycle where things can bog down. Imagine if, when an event happens, something interferes with your ability to work out what you actually feel – is it jealousy or is it mistrust? You may not be able to work out the reasons for why you are feeling the way that you do (step 3). Ultimately, you will not be able to reduce the tension, resulting in confusion. Confusion is just another not-OK feeling. This can cause a cascade of difficulties throughout the rest of the cycle and may result in a range of behaviours from inaction to inappropriate action. Inappropriate action is action that does not work for you or those around you.

If the result is a serious build-up of not-OK feelings, self-worth will plunge. When self-worth deteriorates, many associated areas like physical self-image and male or female self-image will also start dropping. I have included some notes on self-worth in Appendix 1.

All of this emphasises just how important it is to keep these mental lines of communication within the feelings–thoughts–actions cycle working as well as possible. This, as with any mental health difficulty, would be a key area in which to change things.

Naturally, the experience of hearing voices also figures in the cycle.

In this respect, I would like to draw your attention to a single little word in the cycle – 'event'. It is of prime importance in the whole business of hearing voices. When the 'event' cannot readily be associated with what my other senses are telling me, a potential problem arises. What if I am hearing a voice but there is nobody else about?

Let me give you a personal experience to illustrate a similar dilemma that confronted me. It also illustrates Friedrich Nietzsche's statement (1886–7): 'There are no facts, only interpretations.'

It had been a tough morning at work. People were scratchy and a difficult workload was staring me in the face. I needed a break from this electric atmosphere; the staffroom and a cup of tea beckoned. I picked up my cup with spoon in it and set off to the staffroom.

Routledge
Taylor & Francis Group

As I walked down the passage, I soon became aware of a sort of whispering sound. Because I was distracted by the day's happenings and my ruffled feelings I could not easily find a reason for it. This in turn made the sound more important.

The passage contained a number of offices. There was my answer: people were talking in the offices. Immediately, however, there was a problem with this guess: I knew that these offices were certainly not all occupied at the same time, yet the sound remained at a constant volume. It also struck me later that I had at this stage – true to Nietzsche's view – made an assumption about what I was hearing: a voice or voices.

I had to make a second guess and it was again about voices. This time, however, the guess placed the voices behind me at the far end of the passage – making sense of why the sound was constant but low in volume. I stopped and turned around to look. The passage was empty.

I can clearly remember the feelings – panic soon followed by escalating desperation to try to find the cause of these voices. Because I was getting more stressed by my own assumptions on top of the day's discomfort my further guesses became wilder, and I was soon starting to feel very uncomfortable and anxious.

A few moments later a concerted effort at gathering my scattering thoughts revealed that what I was in fact hearing and misinterpreting was the sound of my spoon in my mug – scraping backwards and forwards, in rhythm with my walking.

One of the key processes that played a role here was anxiety. Basically, I had left the room because I was feeling anxious. Anxiety is potentially one of the most destructive feelings that we experience.

None of us are ever without anxiety. You may not feel it acutely, but it is there. This is because no one is ever entirely at ease about the things going on around them or in their head.

The best explanation of anxiety I have heard is when put in relation to fear. When you feel fear the real tiger is standing in front of you. In anxiety, the tiger is in your head; you are thinking about the tiger without it being there in the flesh. That means you cannot run from it or climb a tree. It is this quality of anxiety – the fact that you cannot run from what is going on in your head – that gives it such negative qualities. It leaves you with a feeling of being cornered without being able to see what is cornering you.

Ⓡ Routledge
Taylor & Francis Group

Anxiety has exactly the same effects as fear, ranging from discomfort to reaching a kind of paralysis. You may even faint. It is when anxiety escalates that problems can arise. It differs from fear because of its quality of cornering you and thus meaning that it feeds on itself.

Anxiety is perhaps the biggest culprit among the emotions. It is an emotion with qualities that makes it the thug of emotions right across the mental health spectrum. A summary of its qualities could be:

- There is no obvious or understandable feared object that can be directly addressed.
- Even if the mental 'object' is found, dealing with it is a laborious and fraught process.
- It can be triggered very easily.
- Anxiety escalates rapidly and can move to the point of incapacitating the person.
- It is easily misinterpreted as indicating a bad physical illness (with heart attacks, abdominal cancer and strokes being common misinterpretations), which then, in turn, escalates anxiety further.
- Because the anxious person continually searches for a solution, the anxiety is sustained, thereby keeping the person at an undesirably high level of anxiety for long periods.
- Anxiety can very quickly distort thinking, including perception and concentration, as well as severely disrupting short-term memory.

It is therefore no surprise that we all have difficulty dealing with anxiety effectively. The most common strategy we use is to try to avoid the thoughts that are triggering the anxiety. The negative effects on anxiety of avoidance, particularly repeated avoidance, can be depicted as a graph (see Figure 5).

 Routledge Taylor & Francis Group

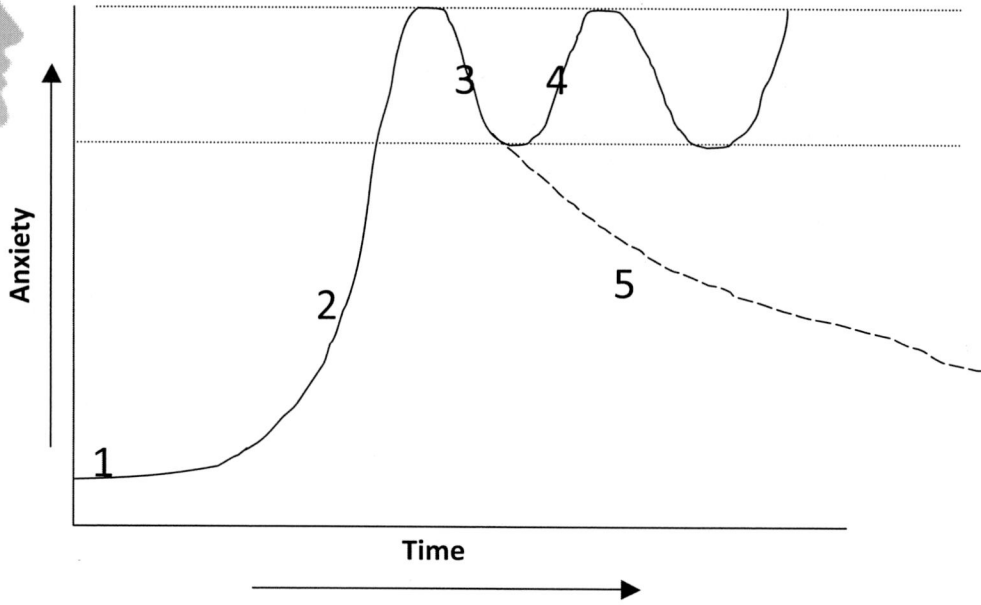

Figure 5   The effect of repeated avoidance on anxiety, adapted from Powell (1992)

Notes

- Point 1 represents the normal level of anxiety.
- When a scary thought enters your mind, anxiety very rapidly gets worse, feeding on itself. It does this by a cycle of more worrying thoughts generating physical symptoms that then increase the stress and anxiety. This escalation is illustrated by the sharply climbing graph, as shown by point 2.
- At point 3 we have applied some form of avoidance, that is, we are not dealing directly with the thought that triggered the anxiety. Our strategy has some effect and the anxiety temporarily drops.
- Because we have not actually dealt with our thoughts that triggered anxiety, it rises again – as indicated at point 4.
- We again apply the temporary solution and produce the zigzag type of graph shown.
- Point 5 shows an interesting phenomenon; if we do nothing, that is, exercise no strategy of avoidance and just stay in the presence of the anxiety, then the anxiety naturally tends to decrease. (This is one of the techniques that therapists use in desensitising people with phobias.)

You will notice a couple of other characteristics about the graph. There are two stipple lines between which the zigzag takes place. This means that anxiety is now hovering between the two lines for an extended period and this level is much higher than where you started at point 1. Avoidance typically causes your anxiety to 'freeze' at that high level.

There is another feature that I have not included in this representation. Somewhere above the zigzag line is another line that represents a threshold. This is the threshold above which point sustained anxiety pushes you towards mental breakdown – being increasingly likely if you often reach these levels of anxiety and remain trapped there for extended periods. Avoidance strategies may well keep anxiety high for extended periods.

All of this strongly suggests that using any kind of avoidance as opposed to dealing with the anxious thought openly and directly is bad news. Avoidance is a very ineffective strategy in dealing with anxiety.

Some typical avoidance strategies are:

- trying to drown out the thoughts with noise, for example, mp3 players, the TV or loud music
- trying to wipe out troublesome thoughts and feelings with alcohol or other substances
- not approaching the thing you are worrying about, for example, a difficult telephone call that may involve a confrontation or going to the dentist
- trying to become 'invisible' in some way, for example, pretending you are not in when that feared knock comes at the door.

The opposite of avoidance is a process called focusing, which I will explain later.

Thus, anxiety needs to be dealt with, and it needs to be dealt with in a way that reduces the anxiety. Think of the feelings–thoughts–actions cycle. The whole anxiety package starts with feeling anxious and then automatically rolls through the thought and action components. The major point here is that in anxiety states you are not in control of this process. This is a major component in not handling voices.

High anxiety is very bad for all of us because it can do any or all of the following:

- It seriously interferes with short-term memory.
- There is a drop off in concentration and therefore your ability to solve problems will drop off as well. Under these conditions it could happen that you could misinterpret common sounds and sights. Because of this, it may contribute to you having unusual experiences that cannot be explained easily. (Professionals call these 'anomalous' experiences.)

Ⓡ Routledge
Taylor & Francis Group

- Thoughts may speed up. Racing thoughts cannot be processed effectively.
- You may place more importance on a variety of things, for example, noise, shadows and tastes. In turn, this will give you an inaccurate personal view of the experience.
- Your mouth could feel dry. If this happens it could change the way that things taste. If usual things start tasting different you may wonder if your food has gone off or even if it has been tampered with.
- Your heart could beat in a different way. This could lead to all kinds of fears about heart problems.
- Also causing concern for anxious people is that breathing may change to quick, shallow breaths. Having no knowledge that this is a normal – although unpleasant – bodily reaction when a person feels threatened may cause this reaction to continue.
- There could also be a range of odd visual effects – for example, tunnel vision or visual distortions – further adding to a growing batch of anomalous experiences.
- Things could get so bad that you may feel nauseous and may even faint.
- You may feel a need to go to the toilet more often.
- You may become sweaty.

This cluster of reactions – even if not coming all together – may leave you physically compromised when you least need it. Of greatest concern is, however, the effect it has on you mentally. Confusion, decreased problem-solving ability, an increase in the amount of anomalous experiences – among other effects – can rattle your self-worth, leaving you feeling vulnerable in the world.

I have laid much emphasis on feelings and, in particular, anxiety, because to my mind the cycle kicks off with feelings. The rest of the cycle is an engine to help the person deal with their emotions and transform them into less threatening thoughts and more productive behaviour.

At the end of the day, if you are aware of this mechanism then you can keep your eye on the whole machine so that it works well for you. In effect, it brings you – the whole person – into sharper focus so that you become more of a known (rather than remaining an unknown) to yourself.

Notes

1   Resilience factors: these are abilities that you have that will help you cope with stress. They are life skills that help you face and deal with adversity.

2   Psycho-social: refers to techniques that approach a problem from both the psychological and social perspectives and, in particular, the way that they interact with each other.

Chapter 2

For voice-hearers

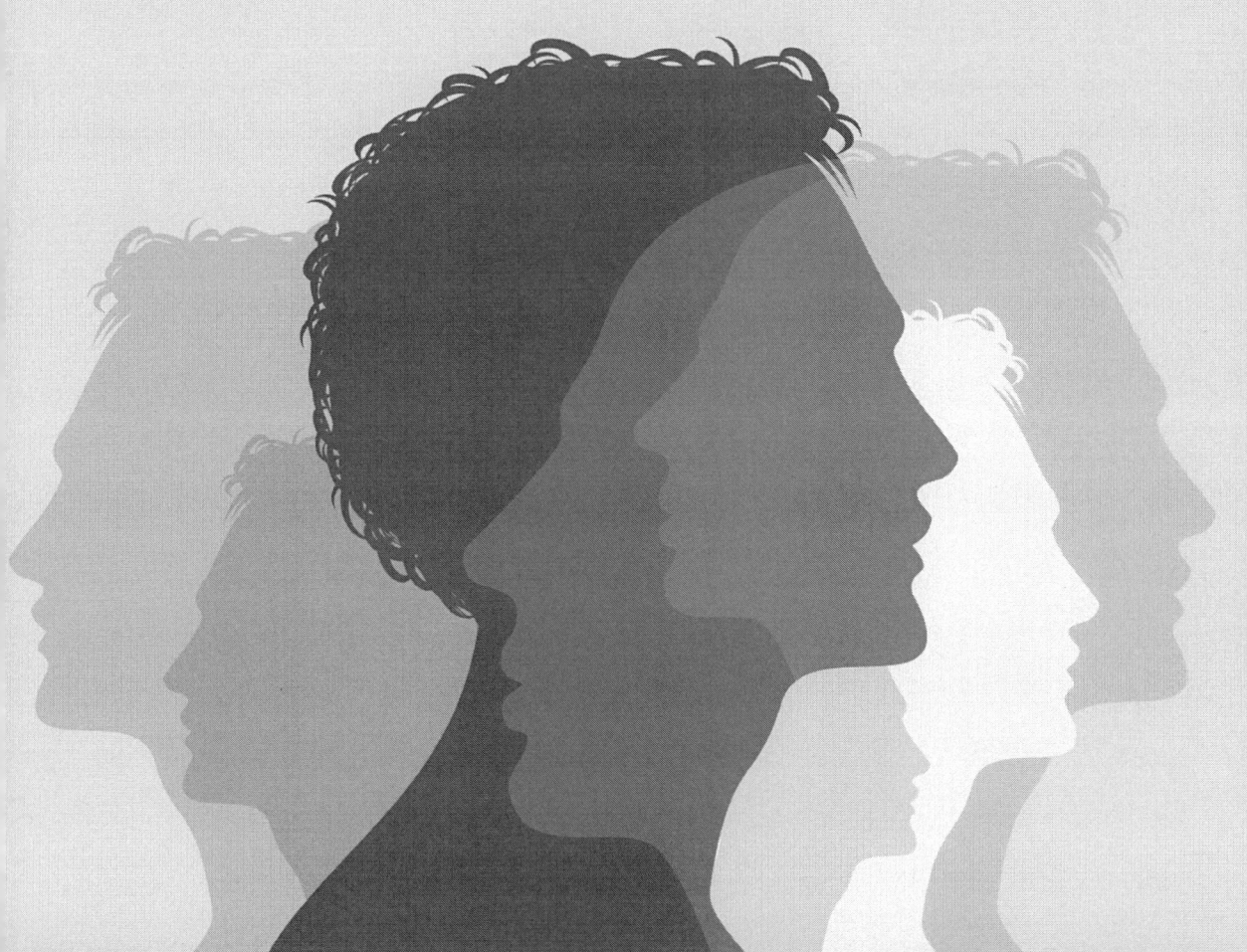

For voice-hearers

2.1 About voices

I had just so many mental problems. It wasn't until I was 28 that my brain actually felt like a spacious place. When I was 18, 19, 22, my brain was just clogged all the time – non-stop voices. I couldn't figure out what was going on. There was a lot of confusion inside me, this flood of voices, often contradicting each other, often telling me stuff that would happen in the future, and then it would happen, voices insulting me, telling me what to do. (Frusciante 2010)

Voices may come in many forms. You may hear the voices of unknown or known individuals. The voices may sound like a person from your past, but this may only strike you later on. There could be more than one voice and even up to 'several hundred', as some clients have reported to me.

Some voices will speak directly to you, whereas others may only comment on what you do. If there are several voices, they may all speak to you in turn or all in a jumble together. They may be talking at you and/or be talking about you.

There could be voices that you believe to be supernatural. Clients have reported these as God, angels, the anti-Christ, Jesus, demons, aliens and others. Please take note that these are all powerful beings. You will see later that your relationship with your voices is based on who has the power in the relationship.

Some clients have also heard the voice(s) of people from powerful but secret organisations like the Central Intelligence Agency (CIA), the Special Branch of the Metropolitan Police or the British Secret Intelligence Service (MI6) and similar.

I have never come across a voice-hearer that hears a voice that is weak. Weak voices will seldom be troublesome. There was one particular voice that one of my clients had that at first glance was a weak voice; it was that of a very young child crying. However, despite it being a child's voice, it was still troublesome. In fact it was hugely distressing to this person because she felt a need to find the crying child. In this sense it caused a major amount of disruption

Routledge
Taylor & Francis Group

in her life. When we hear a crying child we are all drawn to help it. Imagine the torment this person went through not being able to help this child or understand what was making it cry. It was a very powerful, disruptive and troublesome voice indeed.

Surprisingly often people I have worked with can describe their voices as if they can see the people who are talking – although they add that they cannot actually see them. The voice quality conjures up a picture of what the owner of the voice may look like. We all have a similar experience with radio personalities when we do not know what they actually look like; our mind constructs a picture of the face that goes with the voice.

It is fairly common to find that some voices have some of the characteristics of someone you know, but the other characteristics of that person do not in any way fit the character of the voices. For example, a client once said to me that the voice he was hearing sounded like that of an eight year-old but was confused as this child was saying the kinds of things that an adult would say. If you experience something similar and untangle the two qualities – the sound and what they are saying – you may come to understand that the voice is actually mimicking at least two people you knew. You may, for instance, recall that what it is saying reminds you of someone who bullied or abused you, while the quality of the voice sounds like someone else.

I want to stress that the voices I am dealing with all have common features, the most common being that they are distressing. The distress that voices cause is usually intense. Voices seem to know all about you. They seem to be experts on your weaknesses and things you believe you have done wrong or feel guilty about. They bully you. They confuse you. They degrade you. They command you to do things that you would not usually do.

Here are some comments from clients about what their voices do:

- They are there all the time; I am never alone. I can never experience silence.
- They come and go as they please.
- They shout at me.
- They criticise whatever I do and think.
- They curse at me.
- They instruct me to harm myself and/or kill myself.
- They tell me that I am responsible for others' problems and am causing them harm.
- They get louder the more anxious and/or angry and/or depressed I get.

Routledge
Taylor & Francis Group

- They force me to walk in a certain way or move my body in a certain way.
- They wake me up when I am asleep.
- They are there first thing in the morning.
- They continually point out to me how bad and useless or evil I am.
- They know everything I am thinking.
- They are very powerful.
- They move (parts of) my body without my consent.
- They threaten me with punishment or tell me that someone will punish me.
- They talk about me among themselves.

So the picture we have of voices is that they:

- are loud
- come and go when they want to
- are brutal
- are abusive
- are bullying.

Voices are never simple, but one thing is crystal clear: they call the shots in your relationship with them. They have the power. This is our target. This is what must change.

2.2 Things that give your voice power

There are a number of experiences that will help your voices to keep their powerful position in your life. By understanding them you can place these experiences in the right perspective. In this way you are removing some of the tools and weapons that your voices can attack you with.

As hearing voices whips up anxiety, this is one of the things we have to challenge because it plays a huge role in being able to deal with voices and what they do. To tackle any task, anxiety needs to be brought under control.

I have already mentioned anxiety under emotions, thoughts and actions (in section 1.2); however, I would like to expand a bit on it here because it is a difficult feeling to understand. Perhaps it is because we have so many different words and ways of describing it: 'tension', 'stress', 'worry', 'strain', 'pressure' and 'burden' are all words that people may use when they are feeling anxious. For example, people often say, 'I'm feeling stressed.'

R Routledge Taylor & Francis Group

You feel stressed when:

- You have to do something and you don't know how.
- You are not managing because too many things are happening at the same time.
- You are in a bad place and you feel that you can't change anything.
- Nobody is listening to you or hearing what you say.

These are fairly obvious 'bad' scenarios that stimulate anxiety. However, stress can also come with good events; for example:

- You may be enjoying something very much, but you are doing too much of it. This often happens on holiday, for example.
- You are going to have your first child who you have always been wanting, but you are starting to worry about things.
- You have just started your first job.

When you feel you are not coping and the pressure just seems never to stop, you can become very anxious. Also, if the demands that are around seem too big to handle, you can become anxious and confused. Another way we all can get very anxious is when too many demands are happening all at the same time. When anxiety escalates, your concentration drops off and handling problems becomes more difficult.

Remember, too, that you place a lot of demands on yourself! Sometimes we are our own worst enemies.

The solution often lies in going back to the way you say to yourself, 'This is *very important*' or ' I *must* do this *now*' or 'Something *bad* will happen if I don't do it in this way'. I find it useful to question these demands: Why is it *so* important? Why is it something I must do *now*? What is the *bad* thing I fear?

Another dangerous quality of anxiety is that when you are anxious the labels you put on things can be incorrect. When you get very anxious, you can misinterpret ordinary things.

Routledge
Taylor & Francis Group

Misinterpreting normal experiences

In a lot of cases what we experience is just the way the body and mind deal with difficult but normal situations and experiences.

I would like you to look at the following list of experiences. All of us have these from time to time. Many of them can be very unpleasant. These unpleasant experiences can make you very anxious – particularly if you cannot identify what is causing them.

Anxiety is a normal experience but it is unpleasant. Although I have already mentioned the effects of anxiety, it is important to point them out here as well:

- You may easily forget the things you have recently done (your short-term memory drops off).
- Your thoughts may feel quite muddled. Even everyday problems become difficult to handle.
- Some or all of your thoughts may speed up.
- Strangely, things that were never important to you before may now become important. The opposite of this could also happen; things that were important to you now seem unimportant. This may happen to everyday experiences like an increase or decrease in the importance of, for example, noises, shadows and tastes.
- It is quite usual for your mouth to become dry. One of the problems this could then cause is that things may taste different to usual. You could then mistakenly think that somebody has messed with your food.
- Anxiety, like fear, gets your heart to beat in a different way. It may beat faster or more slowly but with deep beats. In cases like this some people could become anxious about the possibility of a heart attack.
- Although you may not be immediately aware of it, your breathing can change to quick shallow breaths.
- Your vision may play tricks, for example, problems in focusing or tunnel vision.
- You could even feel so anxious that you feel like throwing up.
- You may feel the need to go to the toilet more often.
- You could feel hot or cold and quite sweaty.

Apart from anxiety, there are a lot of other normal events that can play into the hands of voices.

Lack of sleep (continual poor sleep) can cause some strange effects.

- If you have regularly been missing out on a lot of sleep the effects can build up over time. Tiredness will increase. A feeling that you are not quite 'with it' may well kick in alongside poor concentration and a drop off in performance.
- When you have had absolutely no sleep for a period of two to four days then experiences could become very strange and it is quite likely that you could start badly misinterpreting things. This is quite common in obvious things like sounds, colours and shapes. Worst of all you may even see and hear things that no one else can see or hear.
- From time to time we all experience disturbing dreams and you can then wake up feeling anxious and tense. You may occasionally have a dream that is so vivid (or scary) that it stays with you throughout the day and may even confuse you.

The time between going to sleep and waking up can be a time of strange experiences.

- It is at times like these that you may experience body jerks and a lot of strange hypnotic, dream-like experiences. They can be unpleasant, pleasant or even creative and helpful in solving problems. They are quite normal.

Automatic negative thoughts pop into our heads and are unpleasant.

- Certain thoughts pop into our heads that are always presenting a negative – and often self-critical – suggestion or description of ourselves. They often centre on failure. We all have them every day. We have become used to them in a way, but they are still unpleasant and can leave you feeling uncertain and perhaps even bad about yourself.

Others around you have an effect on you (called a 'group effect').

- If, for instance, life at home has been filled with mysteries and unspoken threats, you may come to expect that this is the way of the world and become on your guard. Also, if important people around you often show anger and hostility then you may come to believe that all people are angry and hostile. If you have been shielded and over-protected from life you may well come to believe that life is always safe and a walk-over.

Powerful emotions have an effect on us.

- Feelings like anger, fear, love and jealousy can cause your thinking to become quite twisted. When this happens the way you experience things in general may become distorted as well.

We react to major personal loss or trauma.

- Sometimes life dishes you a bolt from the blue that shakes you to the core. When this happens there may be some unpleasant but normal reactions. You can always expect unpleasant reactions to abnormal conditions.

ℝ Routledge
Taylor & Francis Group

Example of the effect of trauma:

This story was brought to my attention by a person I was seeing in therapy and who had a diagnosis of paranoid schizophrenia.

After the terrorist attack on New York on 11 September 2001 (9/11), a story went that a fire fighter was heard to say: 'Sometimes when one experiences trauma, the things that are happening at the same time are not put in your mind at the right place. This leaves one with a confused picture of the event.'

The quote, my client said, reflected closely her own experience but with the difference that her trauma was extended over several years.

Drugs and alcohol have effects.
- The effects of drugs and alcohol are unpredictable. Sometimes withdrawing from drugs can produce as many problems as being on the drugs and, once again, the effects themselves are unpredictable. Drugs and alcohol are really bad news whichever way you look at them.

Intense thinking about the meaning of existence has effects.
- Too much thinking about existence and the meaning of life could easily make life's problems seem worse and more complex. This will pump up anxiety.

We misunderstand emotions and this can have negative consequences.
- Most of us are not skilled in working out what it is that we are feeling and what we should do about it. So sometimes we can mistake jealousy for 'paranoia', loneliness for being disliked by others and so on.

Memories and thoughts can come out of nowhere and be unsettling.
- Your mind is never still. There are many thoughts flying about; most of them you are not aware of. There are automatic negative thoughts, old memories and many other things unsettling the mind. These unconscious thoughts can often be triggered by something small and insignificant. Having an unknown thought just pop into your head can sometimes be quite unsettling. A vague sense of recognition about time, place and person, called déjà vu feelings, often cause a lot of concern. Déjà vu feelings are quite normal. They can, however, leave you feeling worried – as if you have a problem that needs to be solved, but cannot pin down.

 Routledge Taylor & Francis Group

It is very important to know that many of these normal experiences can be misinterpreted. Often, people who hear voices tie these misinterpretations to their voices. Should you believe that your voices are causing these, it will make the voice seem all the more powerful.

> *Be careful not to give your voice any power. When you think that it has qualities that it does not actually have, you are giving it power.*

2.3 The first step: changing the way that you think about voices

The first steps I am asking you to take are really a way of preparing the stage for your campaign against your voices. Without this preparation, it is not going to fly.

It is thus very important that you think about the following:

- **You are in a relationship with your voices.** Because your voice often conveys a message to you that is more or less understandable and you are able to act on that message in some way, this makes what is happening sound very much like a relationship. The next point takes this definition a step further.
- **These are your voices; nobody else has them.** Other voice-hearers have voices that may be similar but when you get to the detail, they are exclusive to a particular voice-hearer. Just like a circle of work colleagues or even friends that are exclusively yours, your voices are exclusively yours.
- **Treat the voices as if they are 'real' people**, however crazy this sounds. Remember that this is only 'as if'. You do this to help you understand that you actually have a relationship with them. Only then can you deal with the problems they present to you, as you would with a flesh and blood person.
- **Some people cope with their voices**; it is possible for you to learn to cope with yours as well.
- **Voices are not superpowerful.** If voices were that powerful then nobody would be able to cope with them and nobody would learn how to cope with them.

To help you with changing the way that you think about voices, imagine that you have a friend who is being bullied at work. How would you advise them to respond to the bully? Have a look at these options. Would you tell your friend to:

- ignore the bully?
- start bullying back – playing the same game?
- call on the help of a more powerful person?
- look for another job?
- keep quiet and keep a stiff upper lip and take it?
- have a drink in order to calm down?

Getting back to you, most often your voices are bullying you in some way. If you gave yourself advice about what to do, would you tell yourself to:

- try to ignore your voice(s)?
- shout, scream and swear at them?
- call on the help of a more powerful person?
- move to another house or town because maybe your voice will not come with you?
- grin and bear it?
- start abusing substances to calm yourself and the voice down?

If you do not think that any of these are such a good idea, why not? Ask yourself:

- Will any of these actions stop the bully?
- Will any of these actions change the fact that perhaps you allow yourself to be bullied?

All of the suggestions above have got something in common:

- They all avoid the issue: you keep allowing yourself to be victimised.
- They support the bully and give him or her satisfaction and power.
- You will remain a victim. (Put another way, you probably are still seen by your bully and perhaps others as a victim.)
- You keep your self-worth low *or* you may have it damaged further.
- It's a lost opportunity for learning
  - about dealing with bullies in general
  - assertive behaviour
  - that you *can* be equal.

I should not allow myself to be dominated or controlled by anyone.

Avoiding a problem does not solve it.

The key question that comes out of the above is: How do you get back to being equal with your voice? I am also referring to how to get equal in any relationship; there is no reason why you should treat your voices any differently. Your voice cannot be allowed to:

- call the shots
- tell you what to do and how to do it
- turn up at any time and expect you to drop everything to listen to what it has to say
- threaten you
- curse at, swear at and abuse you without a response.

However, your voice can be allowed to:

- have an opinion
- make suggestions
- give you health warnings
- talk to you in a calm way
- approach you rather than gatecrash.

Your response to your voice should not be aggressive; it is more about being assertive – regaining the initiative and regaining choice.

The *Dorland's Medical Dictionary* (2015) says that assertive behaviour contains the following parts. It:

- is a confident statement by you without you needing to prove it
- identifies your rights or point of view
- is not aggressive or threatening

- does not deny the rights of the other person
- does not allow the other person to ignore your rights or point of view.

> **I should be firm but not aggressive when dealing with a bully, or indeed anyone.**

By now you are probably coming to understand that the relationship you have with your voice has a lot, if not everything, to do with power. It is a relationship in which you:

- see your voice as powerful
- see yourself as weaker
- have developed a great fear of your voice(s).

In the first chapter I mentioned that Professor Marius Romme discovered three phases in the progress of the voice-hearing relationship. The first phase he called the 'startling phase'. This is when you first hear voices and you become startled. What I have not yet mentioned is that many people who hear voices become stuck in the startling phase. Being startled is a type of fear response. In other words, each and every time your voice arrives, you are startled and experience fear. Why do you think that this is?

A psychiatrist I once knew had a very interesting saying: 'If you keep putting your head in the sand, you will get your butt kicked!' That is very true.

> **If you keep denying that you hear a voice, you will know nothing about it; it will remain a stranger and every time it pitches up you will be startled.**

Moving this one step further, we can say: the more we get to know about something, the less we will fear it. This counts for everything we come across: from knowing how your new kettle works right up to knowing how to use a computer.

> **When I get to know about something, I fear it less.**

Routledge
Taylor & Francis Group

2.4 The second step: getting to know your voices

You can gather information about your voice by using the following questions. This is often called a 'Voice Profile'. Write down your answers for each voice you hear:

- **Is your voice male or female?** If you have no idea, then ask your voice. If it remains quiet then you decide if it is a male or a female and then address it accordingly. It may then try to correct you, so then you will have your answer. If it says nothing, then stick with your decision until it does correct you. If it keeps chopping and changing its mind about this, then you decide and stick to your decision.

- **What is your voice's name?** If your voice has not given you its name, then ask him or her, as you would any stranger. If they do not answer, give them another chance; ask again. If there is still no response, you could think of naming the voice yourself. It is best to avoid giving your voice a powerful name like 'God' or 'Satan'; rather give it a neutral name. Remember this name and stick to it. If your voice then later comes up with another name, negotiate with it. Do not accept a powerful name or one that scares you. Remember, in a relationship the one who calls the shots is in control. So, a voice coming back and saying 'My name is Beelzebub' will be calling the shots, unless of course you say to him or her that you will consider it. You have to get into the driving seat whenever possible.

- **Does your voice remind you of someone?** Can you conjure up a mind's eye picture of your voice? If not, you can think about 'interviewing' your voice by asking it a few questions about itself. If your voice does not answer, do not pursue this strategy; a person who only produces silence is also controlling. However, you may tell it that you will return to the question at a later time. Then return with the questions at a later time. If it still does not answer, then drop the subject. If it later volunteers information, thank it. If the information sounds ridiculous, question it.

- **What does your voice say to you? Write it down.** This is a bit like you becoming a press reporter. If you don't understand something it says, interrupt it and ask a question. Again, they may not answer but by interrupting it you have taken some control back. Always think in terms of regaining control and power.

- **Jot down the history of your voice-hearing.** When did it first happen? What was happening at about that time in your life or in the year before that? Is there anything that seems to bring it on or make it worse, or better? In this way you can learn a lot about what triggers your voice and this gives you another tool to limit the time in your life that it occupies. You may also learn about some tricks you have been using that hamper your voice.

Routledge Taylor & Francis Group

- **What is your voice feeling? What does it sound like?** We all show our feelings in the way we speak. Maybe your voice sounds angry? But perhaps it is not actually angry. Listen again. Ask it if it is angry. If you think it sounds angry, say so. 'I think you sound angry.'

- **Does your voice laugh and do you think it's laughing at you?** Think about this: why do people laugh? Sometimes people laugh because they feel embarrassed, and don't know what to say. Sometimes people laugh at an inner joke. Are you still sure the voice is laughing *at* you? Are you in fact sure it is laughter? Sometimes people sound as if they are laughing but they are really crying.

- **Is there any particular time when your voice comes?** Does your voice come more often in certain circumstances; perhaps it comes when you feel certain emotions like anger or fear or anxiety? Maybe you could keep a little diary.

- **How long does it stay, usually?** Minutes? Hours? Days? Is there perhaps something you do (or do not do) that really keeps it going or, on the other hand, that shortens the time it stays or how often it comes?

- **Is it always abusive and is that abuse always directed at you?** Many of us swear when we are frustrated or angry or even when we are sad and downhearted. Often when we do this it is not directed at anyone in particular. You need to consider this; possibly you are not the target.

- **Is there anything that you have done that gets it to change in any way?** For example, you may find that when you do certain things or say certain things it gets worse or it quietens down, or becomes more or less abusive. Some people have even reported that the voice itself may change into another, perhaps friendlier, voice.

- **Does your voice speak clearly?** If your voice mumbles then ask it (nicely) to speak more clearly. Of course, it may not do as you ask, but the point is that you have spoken up.

- **Does your voice make any mistakes?** If your voice says something that makes no sense, question it. If it is making a downright mistake, point it out. If it starts arguing with you, don't get dragged into the argument. It is your choice what you do.

> *Getting to know your voice is like creating a map so that you can see what you are dealing with.*

You will notice that a lot of the above includes talking to your voice. I know that sounds very strange; I have been told that by many a voice-hearer. The problem is that keeping quiet in a situation where you are being verbally dominated means that you are the underdog.

> *Keeping quiet could mean that you agree with what the voice is saying.*

It is better to try to strike up some kind of a dialogue.[1] Even if your voice still does not respond to you, at least you are not lying down and taking it.

> *The more you stand up and face your voice, the better you will feel within yourself – even if your knees are shaking.*

You may even start feeling that the voice is not that powerful any more, purely due to the fact that you are standing up for yourself and talking back. Please remember: be calm, but assertive. Like any bully, voices would love you to get wound up. Do not give them that satisfaction.

There is an interesting event that most voice-hearers I have worked with report back to me with some consternation. They say: 'I talked to my voice. I asked it why it kept bothering me, but it did not answer me. The technique has not worked!'

> *Your voice does not have to answer you. If your voice does not answer, maybe it does not have an answer.*

Remember, you are treating your voice as if it is a real person, and real people do not have to answer you. This is not about forcing a response out of your voice; it is about you standing up and doing something. You are not trying to become the bully; you are in fact changing your position in the relationship from being passive to being active.

2.5 The third step: paying attention to your self-worth

When your voice is around, you really have to take extra care of your self-worth and self-respect. I will describe this in more detail later (also see Appendix 1)

We all carry a view of ourselves with us all the time and everywhere. A trustworthy view of yourself will help you through many important life situations. However, your self-worth can get undermined quite easily, particularly if you hear voices.

Routledge
Taylor & Francis Group

Imagine if someone kept making remarks about your hair – you may well start believing that there was something wrong with your hair. All of us react like this. The constant negative remarks seem to sink in and, before you know it, you will be thinking like that. Constant criticism by a voice will lead you towards criticising yourself. This is a good reason to challenge the critical or abusive voice.

One of the reasons that this happens to all of us from time to time is because basically none of us feel OK about ourselves. It is very easy for us to find fault with ourselves. Mostly we are not aware of this somewhat negative picture we carry around about ourselves. Then, someone comes along and seems to hit on something we may feel bad about, responsible for or sensitive about. Voices are experts at this.

> **Voices find and highlight your weaknesses, fears and faults.**

I sometimes think that perhaps voices are, in a strange way, like a teacher that lets you look at the things you have been avoiding looking at. These are the things that we all keep on the back shelf in our minds: the memories and thoughts we do not like dealing with. Perhaps voices are saying that these need to be looked at and fixed. But I am only speculating here.

All of this means that if you and I had a self-worth that was OK, perhaps we would not be so bothered by what anyone, including voices, say to us and about us.

In section 1.2 I described self-worth with a few points that I will repeat here.

- Self-worth is what I think about myself.
- It is not what others think of me; that's why it's called *self*-worth.

My self-worth depends on:

- recognising when I get something right
- saying 'thanks' to myself from time to time
- saying 'hello' to myself from time to time
- recognising my achievements, however small
- asking myself what I want from time to time
- praising myself when it's due

- looking for the good in me
- daring to be myself
- putting myself equal to (not above or below) others
- not always criticising myself
- taking actions to try to fix it when I find fault with something that I have done
- accepting that others may be different to me but that they are not really better than I am
- treating myself with respect.

Thus, when your voices are telling you how bad you are, over and over again, you may start believing that what your voice says is true, but if you have built up a more worthy picture of yourself then you will know that this is not the truth. Just like if a person makes a remark about your hair, your hand-writing or the way you walk, you will know it is just a remark – just an opinion – and not the truth. It is you who holds the truth about yourself, not your voices.

I remember telling my wife many times about how concerned I was becoming about the way one of my work colleagues was continually trying to put me down in clinical meetings. I still remember her response, 'Why are this person's remarks so important to you?' She was right; I did not even like or respect this person. Now I am asking you the same question:

Why are your voice's remarks so important to you?

I was, in some way, making my work colleague's critical remarks important and, similarly, you are probably making your voice's remarks important to you.

Eventually, I just let him rave on without attaching importance to what he was saying. I just said to myself: 'Oh, that's him popping off again.' This is of course easier said than done, but when he did not get the usual defensive response from me, after a while his remarks ground to a halt. He was playing the game called 'I will attack you, and you will defend', which really is a set of instructions. He was sucking me into something I did not want to be part of. As soon as I started defending myself, the game was on and he had in fact won.

Don't play the game that your voice suggests.

Ⱳ Routledge
Taylor & Francis Group

It is also important to realise:

> *Every time you find just one instance when you are not as bad as the voice is saying, you are also finding an instance when your voices are wrong.*

That means that if the voices are wrong sometimes, they cannot be all that powerful, can they? It also means that if the voices cannot get you to do everything they want you to do, then who is running the show?

If you want to create and retain an OK self-worth, you need to remind yourself all the time of these discoveries about your voices. At the end of the day, it is also about self-respect.

> *Start treating yourself with respect; perhaps the voices will also do that.*

I mentioned above that there are times when I was with the critical colleague and I just let him rave on; I let it run off my back. Before I got this right I had to correct two things I was doing:

1 I was listening out and waiting for his criticisms. I was expecting them and this made me very tense.
2 While I was 'waiting' for these criticisms, I found it difficult to get on with the usual things in my day.

I had to stop doing both of these.

> *Listening and waiting for a scary thing will make you anxious.*

With regards to point 1, let me point out a very common thing we all do and, as such, is often done by voice-hearers: selective listening. Selective listening can be used both for and against you. Listening out for your voice is an example of where you are using it to work against you. Alternatively, we all use it to work for us without knowing it — as in the example below:

> When you go to the supermarket, your mind is busy with many things besides getting your shopping done. Perhaps you don't like being among people. Perhaps you are trying to remember if you locked your door. Perhaps you are worried about how long the shopping is taking and that you may miss your bus. There is also a lot of noise in the shop. Although

R Routledge
Taylor & Francis Group

you are aware of these things, your mind gets on with the job of shopping; it does not allow any of these to interfere to the extent that you cannot get any shopping done.

Somehow, your mind puts all of these questions into the background. It does so by making the present task more important than the others; it finds a reason to make the present task more important. Perhaps it is possible that, because of the fear attached to voices, you make the noise that the voices produce too important? Maybe trying to do the opposite – that is, making something else more important – is what you could aim for? Of course it takes practice, but if you get it right once, you can do it again.

> **There are other things that are more important than your voices.**

I remember a client telling me that despite her voices ranting at her, when her horse started foaling, she said to her voices: 'I cannot listen to you now; I have to help my horse first.' She helped her horse in spite of the presence of the voices.

2.6 Special tricks

Using the 'in spite of' attitude

As you become more active in the relationship with your voices, you can consider introducing some tricks that are proactive as well. This means that instead of waiting for your voices to do something and then reacting, you can do something before your voices arrive. Reacting is what a puppet does when someone pulls the string. A puppet is out of control because it is reacting.

This proactive trick tries to neutralise something that you fear will happen or is definitely going to happen. However, we all forget that most things, even the bad things, come to an end. If you can realise this in any situation – for example, going to the dentist, a difficult interview or an exam – it takes some of the sting out of the event. The trick I use (and it calms me down every time) is to say to myself: 'In two hours' time the (bad) thing will be over.' This tells me that the distress will end; it will not go on forever. In many cases this is also true of your voices; at some point your voices will be quieter or even give you a break. (Imagine if you had a set of tricks to organise that as well!)

Routledge
Taylor & Francis Group

With practice, the tactic can play a positive role even when the voices are present. In our early intervention team we talked of the 'in spite of' strategy. What this means is that you carry on with your life *in spite of* the presence of the voices. This may not be that easy when you start working on your voices but it will be a useful tool later as you get more control.

> **The 'in spite of' strategy says: I am not going to let what is happening now ruin my day.**

Lying to your voices

Although this trick is not really proactive it is so unexpected that it could get the voice off your back; it feels like you are doing something entirely new with your voices. Lying may not sit easily with you but in the relationship with your voices it is allowed.

In the voice-hearers group we ran we discovered that one of the voice-hearers was actually doing this without knowing he was doing it. The situation was that ever so often his voice would give him clear instructions to harm himself. As many voice-hearers follow the command, it struck my colleague and I that he never attempted it. When asked why there was this difference, he explained that when the command came he told the voice he would do it, but he just never did. In other words what he said and what he did were different. He was lying to his voice. When I pointed this out to him, he looked guilty. His guilty feeling illustrates the power he felt the voice had; he felt bad because he was not doing what his voice had told him to do. I added that there was nothing wrong with this type of lie. The effect of this lie on the voice was that it left him immediately for that moment. He had scored a point on his voice. It is also interesting that another member of the group tried this strategy, which also worked for her. It was not a permanent solution, but it showed these voice-hearers that they could do something that made the voice change what it was doing, even if just for a few hours. If I can make a vicious dog change what it is doing – even for a short time – I have created some control in the relationship.

> **You do not have to do what your voice tells you to do, even if you tell your voice that you will do it. What you do is your choice.**

Making a request of your voice

To many voice-hearers this one sounds very scary because they really just want to leave their voice alone, as if it were a vicious dog. However, we all know that the main reason for the dog being vicious is because it has not been trained. When you train a dog to listen to you, you always do so with a 'softly, softly approach' and without abuse – so too with voices.

Routledge Taylor & Francis Group

Remember, this is not really an instruction you are giving your voice; it is a request. Instructions are an attempt to dominate, which you should not try with voices, or anyone for that matter. Remember, too, requests can be refused or ignored.

> **If your voice does not do what you request, you have not failed.**

Once again, the point here is that you are busy normalising your relationship with your voice. You are not trying to get the voice to do what you tell it to do. Normalising just means changing the relationship in a way that it becomes more like a normal relationship in which no one is abused, controlled or dominated.

Here are some examples of requests:

- When your voice gatecrashes or demands that you have to say or do something right now, ask it to come back at another time. There is nothing aggressive or uncooperative about this. I often had to do this with colleagues when I was at my desk writing a report and someone would just walk up to me and start a conversation. 'Sorry, I'm busy right now; can we talk later?' was all I needed to say. Your voice will probably not just keep quiet; it is a bully, remember. However, what you are trying to do here is to assert yourself and your current needs, which are to finish what you are doing now. You are also taking the other's needs into consideration by suggesting that you will come back to that person later. This follows directly on to the next example.

- When your voice is not around, ask it to come and have a chat. This is probably one of the most proactive strategies you could use and, thus, for most voice-hearers is one of the scariest. However, if you tie it to the previous example, you can, when you are ready, normalise the relationship again; after all, you did say you would get back to the voice. Thus, you can follow up the above at a later stage by saying to your voice that you are now available to talk. There is a very interesting thing that some voice-hearers have expressed after they have tried this strategy. They say: 'I asked my voice to come and it did not come. I have failed.' This is similar to the example I gave of: 'If your voice does not do what you request, you have not failed.' But there is an added point for you here. It is called 'paradoxical intention'. This just means getting what you want by asking for the opposite. Just think about that for a while; people are using this trick all the time. In arguments between people they may say: 'OK, don't talk to me then!' We have all probably said that at some time. If your

Routledge
Taylor & Francis Group

voice does not come when you ask it to, you have actually applied paradoxical intention. You have asked it to come, and it did not come. That's exactly what you want, isn't it? Perhaps your voice does not like you 'telling' it what to do.

What is your voice really trying to tell you?

This is also a proactive strategy and falls into a category that we call existential. This really just means that you are thinking about why you actually hear a voice and if it is perhaps trying to tell you something important. I have touched on this before but not as a proactive strategy. There is a good reason behind this strategy.

> **Whatever we experience has some personal meaning for us.**

Right at the beginning of the book I used the simple example of a single word – 'apple' – and how it had a host of different meanings for me. A single word will bring up different memories, feelings, needs and thoughts for each one of us. Complex experiences like hearing voices may also carry a host of personal meanings. It is not impossible that what your voices say may have a personal meaning for you.

Sometimes we have experiences that we would rather not review and not do anything about; they were too painful or horrific. Our minds have a neat but ultimately unproductive technique for dealing with these experiences. It is quite a child-like technique. When a very young child plays 'Hide and Seek' he or she hides by closing their eyes. The 'reasoning' behinds this is: 'If I cannot see you, you cannot see me.'

Seen in terms of the cycle of feelings–thoughts–actions (Chapter 1), the experience is being sent back into the thought part. It is being filed in a folder that is called 'not me'. So, you try to make your bad experiences invisible; you find a place right in the corner on one of the back shelves of your mind and you hide the experience there. It does not work; eventually those memories will come back, often in the wrong place, at the wrong time and very often in a distorted or symbolic form. This just means that it comes out in a type of a code in which the meaning is unclear to you and others.

Among my clients I have found many cases in which hearing voices has links with some form of social, physical or psychological trauma. In these cases the voice-hearer's mind has made links between what voices are saying, how they sound and the situation that existed at that time.

Routledge
Taylor & Francis Group

It would seem that the voices are often replaying threatening, abusive and dominant elements that were present within the traumatic experience. However, the mind finds this experience too difficult to handle so it pushes it away by representing it as a voice.

What your voice is saying, who it sounds like and the situations that trigger it may well be linked to personal traumatic experiences in your life.

Previously I mentioned a client who discovered that his voice sounded like his father but was saying things that his father would never say. Further investigation revealed a caring but controlling father who ultimately wanted his son to do things his way. What also came up was that in his teens he had been bullied in a very abusive way by a boy in his class. Once these connections could be cleared up, his voices' intrusive nature decreased.

Another, quite religious, client also displayed this mix and match of events and voices. Among other bad experiences, she had been raped by a trusted friend at night. At the same time there had been two classmates who had taken it on themselves to make her life a misery. Does it surprise you to hear that her numerous voices included a god-like but mocking voice and two 'shadowy male figures' who said very little but who she experienced as very threatening? All her bad experiences had become jumbled up and presented in a symbolic way.

Although making these links may be meaningless on the one hand, on the other they could have a significant impact on how you experience your voices.

Having a clearer picture of the personal things that drive your life could help you to have more control in many areas.

These kinds of special tricks will help to normalise the voice-hearing experience for you. They are in fact the everyday rules of how to deal more effectively with people who you are attempting to apply to your voices. Thus, there is nothing really strange or magical about the rules.

In this respect, and as with all things in life, there are some 'don't's'.

Routledge
Taylor & Francis Group

Some 'don'ts' and what to do instead

Although I have mentioned these I would like to stress that many of the voice-hearers I worked with clearly stated that the following responses really do not work at all:

- **Swearing and cursing at the voices.** In most cases the voices just get worse.

- **Keeping quiet (and getting anxious).** Getting anxious quite often makes the voices worse.

- **Pleading with the voices.** Pleading could make you feel quite bad about yourself. It may even make you angry at yourself.

- **Responding with single words.** Sometimes it's like the voices don't hear anything but a full sentence. Responding to them with a single word may not be enough; a dialogue is necessary.

- **Doing what the voices tell you to do.** This puts them in the driver's seat. Many voice-hearers think that if they do what the voices want them to do then the voices will go away or at least leave them alone. Unfortunately, this is not true.

- **Turning up the volume of the TV or MP3 player.** As soon as these such devices are turned off, most voice-hearers I have worked with report that the voices come back, at times sounding even louder than before.

> *Voices love it when you crank up your emotions.*

Instead, you could try to:

- **Remain as calm as possible.** Do not get worked up; if you get wound up, so will your voices.
- **Start a conversation.** Saying 'Go away!' or 'Rubbish!' will not do much to change the relationship you have with your voices. Your attempt should be a full sentence. You will get better at this the more you practice.
- **Respond immediately.** Practice having a few things to say to your voices so that you do not give them time to overwhelm you.
- **Repeat your response to your voices several times.** Do not expect them to hear everything you say; they are not waiting for you to talk, so they will probably miss some of the things you say.
- **Be firm** but not abusive.

R Routledge
Taylor & Francis Group

- **Be unaffected by a silent voice.** A voice going silent may make you angry, frightened and tense. Try not to let that get you down or let yourself feel threatened. Remember, silence can mean many different things. Can you think of a few different things that silence can mean?
- **Remain calm if your voices talk back to you.** Pick up the conversation with them. Don't let them rule you. Keep talking to them until you decide you want to do something else.
- **Say something to them if they just turn up without your permission.** You may want to say something to them like: 'I can't talk with you now because I want to get on with ...'

If any of your tricks do not work the first time, do not despair. Keep practising; never give up! Be patient.

> **Although you may feel like throwing in the towel, never give up.**

2.7 Summary of voice-hearers section

- Hearing voices is unpleasant. In this book I focus on troublesome voices.
- Voices may come in many forms.
- Many people hear voices. Some people do not cope and some cope.
- Treat your voices as if they are real people.
- Many of the things you do around your voices gives them power; you can change that.
- Anxiety is a normal but unpleasant experience.
- It is usual to misinterpret things when you are anxious.
- You are in a relationship with your voices. All of the rules of a normal relationship also apply here.
- Avoiding a problem does not solve it.
- If you keep denying that you hear a voice, you will know nothing about it. It will remain a stranger and every time it pitches up you will be startled.
- You should be firm but not aggressive when dealing with a bully, and indeed anyone.
- When you get to know about something, you fear it less.
- Get to know your voices.
- Keeping quiet could mean that you are agreeing with what the voice is saying.
- The more you stand up and face your voice, the better you will feel within yourself – even if your knees are shaking.

 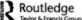

- Pay attention to your self-worth; treat yourself with respect.
- Voices find and highlight your weaknesses, fears and faults.
- Don't play the game that your voice suggests.
- Do not curse at, swear at or scream at your voices; they are better at being abusive in these ways than you are.
- You do not have to do what your voice tells you to do. What you do is your choice.
- Even if they do not listen, try hard to talk to and reason with your voices; it is important to stand up to them.
- However strange it sounds, remember that it is possible that your voice is trying to tell you something personally important.

Notes

1 Dialogue: dialogue is a conversation or discussion. It is more than just one or two words.

Chapter 3

For clinicians

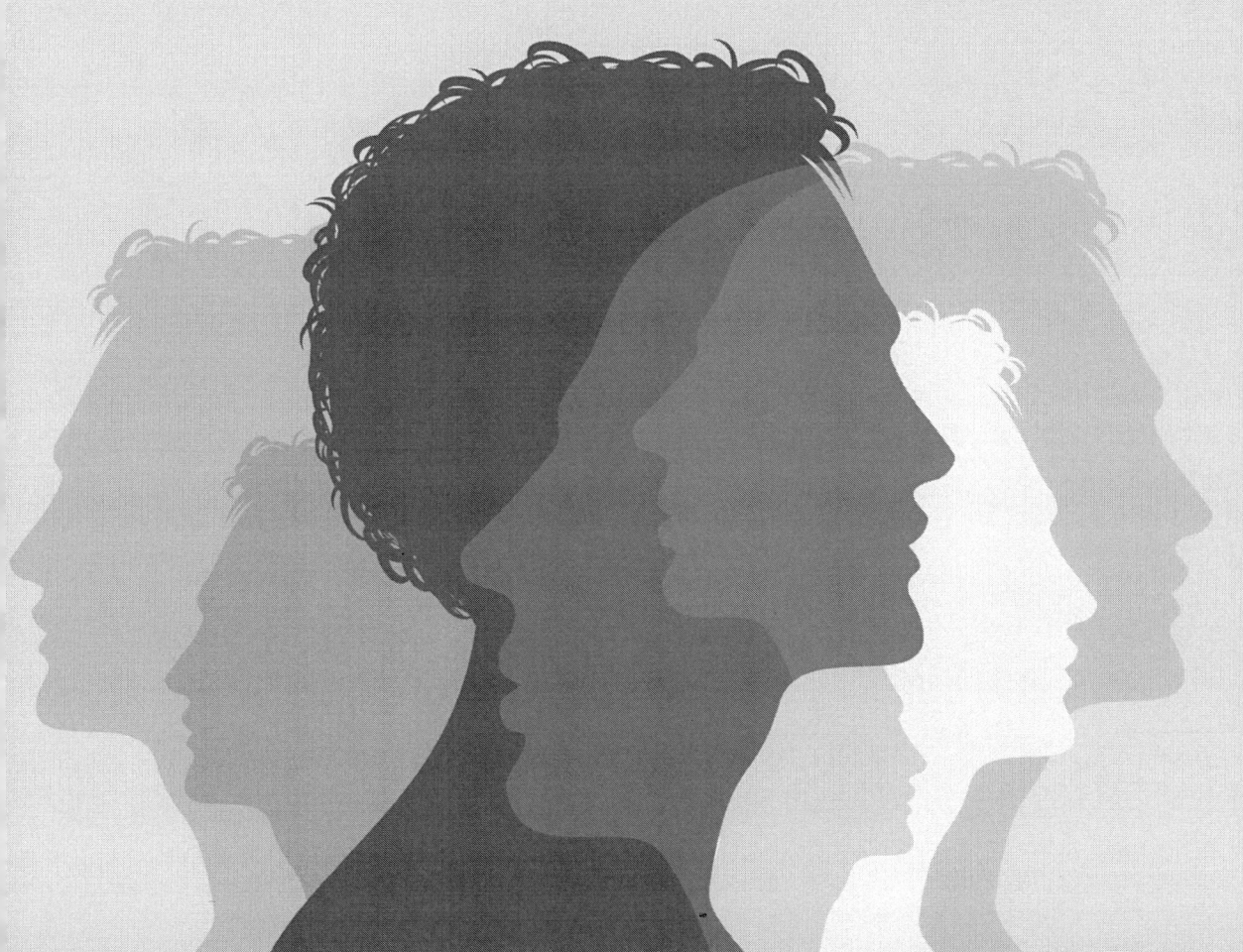

For clinicians

As a clinician, you may ask yourself why you should review the way that you work with voice-hearers. You may even feel somewhat surprised that I have included this section in the book.

When I initially became interested in addressing the whole issue of working with people who hear voices, naturally I needed to find out what people were already doing in this area. The sad truth, I soon learned, was that clinicians had a substantial gap in their skills armoury in this area that would repeatedly place them and their clients in very difficult – if not risky – situations. I also learned that many a clinician was very apprehensive about working with voice-hearers because of a lack of confidence that resulted from their lack of skills. Another, perhaps even more troublesome cause, was voiced by some clinicians; in their core training they were told that they should not attempt any work with the voices of voice-hearers.

After gearing myself up over about a six-month period, I probed these concerns by developing and running a brief training course for ward staff – the aim being to assist ward staff to change their view of voice-hearing and thus to change the way they worked with voice-hearers.

Its broad aims were to:

- develop a practical understanding of the power dynamics inherent in relationships and be able to see how this understanding can be applied to the relationship the voice-hearer has with their voices
- encourage assertiveness techniques to be applied by the voice-hearer in their relationship with their voices; staff would therefore need to understand and encourage assertiveness in the way the client deals with their voices
- encourage client-centredness as a way of staff operating in a relationship (collaborative techniques)
- drive cognitive and cognitive behavioural therapy techniques: with respect to the former, this was to develop a broad understanding of the way in which information is processed, and specifically how delusional characteristics may develop and, further, how such beliefs are maintained; with respect to the latter, this was to develop, specifically, a working knowledge of focusing strategies and how they differ from avoidance strategies and assisting staff in guiding clients in the use of these techniques

 Ⓡ Routledge
Taylor & Francis Group

- drive a narrative approach to investigate the story around the person's voice-hearing experience.

An overall positive outcome highlighted another pressing need: to see if voice-hearers could be helped in a group so that they could learn strategies that worked for them from us as well as from one another.

It was decided to run a group for voice-hearers as an open group in which clients would be encouraged to remain as long as they could but were never contracted to remain for a specific period. It ran thus over a six-year period, during which up to twenty ward-based clients had some taste of a new approach to dealing with their voices. The main aim of the group was to change the experience of hearing voices by:

1 addressing the power and control dynamics inherent in the relationship between voice-hearer and their voice(s)
2 so that the person could move from a position of disempowerment to a position of equality and empowerment in this relationship.

The group was initially based on the work of Romme and Escher (2000) and included the approaches of Irvin Yalom (1975) in his seminal work with groups.

Although voice-hearers in the group found the process stressful they also reported positive effects. They reported:

- being more able to control their voices, resulting in decreased volume and frequency of the experience

- a reduction in intrusive thoughts

- a change in their perception of the threat potential of the voices; voices more often than not seemed less threatening with respect to both the content of their messages and the quality and delivery of the message

- a reduction in, and even a cessation of, self-harming behaviour

- carer reports of substantial reduction in self-harming behaviour and increase in assertive behaviour

- agoraphobic tendencies reduced by regular attendance at group

- that where voices had been heard constantly throughout the day, there were now breaks in the experience due to use of strategies

Routledge
Taylor & Francis Group

- an incorporation of psychological strategies by clients into their dealings with their voices

- that 'standing up to' voices was becoming additional practice in several clients

- greater self-confidence apparent in several clients

- 'cross-pollination' of strategies occurring.

The indications from the initial ward staff training as well as the group for voice-hearers suggested that more staff training was necessary. Together with an occupational therapist (OT) a six-week course was developed. It was delivered across the board to clinicians and was presented to several groups of clinicians over several months.

Apart from the staff showing a clearer understanding of the merits of another approach as well as attempting to actually use it, a striking outcome was that staff felt more empowered in themselves to deal with voice-hearers. They all had moved away from suggesting the client use avoidance (distraction) techniques and towards focusing strategies. They had a new tool in their kit.

> *It would seem that:*
>
> - *A clinician who feels inadequate when working with a certain condition is in an extremely difficult if not depressing situation.*
> - *A clinician who has no techniques to hand will grasp at anything.*

3.1 What should I do?

As a clinician, dealing with voice-hearers – particularly for the first time – is a daunting thought. Luckily, Romme (1998) has provided us with readymade goals for productive work with voice-hearers. These outcomes, for which we should strive, are no less than his findings on the differences between those who hear voices and cope and those who hear voices and do not cope. This must take place against his other powerful advice, and can be summarised as follows:

> *We should stop doing things that do not work or that make things worse.*
> *We should start doing things that move towards an outcome of the person coping with their voices.*

Routledge
Taylor & Francis Group

As a reminder, here is the picture of people who cope (thus defining the goals).

- **People who cope with their voices have proved, and therefore know, that the voices are not so powerful.** The key concept and target here is thus the power difference between the voice-hearer and the voice. View voices as bullies and the voice-hearer as a victim of these bullies. It is your aim to correct this imbalance, helping the voice-hearer to develop a way of dealing with these bullies. As we know, getting worked up or abusive with bullies merely plays into their game. One of the targets is thus to help the voice-hearer to stop this process.

- **People who cope with their voices can see their voices in a different light.** Among others they are able to recognise 'positive' voices. Remember what Friedrich Nietzsche (1886–7) said: 'There are no facts, only interpretations.' Remember, too, that we all define our experiences as OK, neutral or not-OK. If Nietzsche and a lot of others are right about all experience, being interpretations, then the description of certain voices being 'bad' is also an interpretation. Your job then is to change this interpretation by your client. The aim is not to change it into 'My voice is good' but rather to reduce or erode the degree of 'badness' that the voice-hearer attaches to their experience. The shift in perception in effect challenges the voice-hearer's belief that this and all voices are bad. Should you both discover one of their voices that is not that bad or, in the case of a single voice, something that it does that is not that bad or that can be reframed as something neutral or even helpful, then you have made a crack in the wall.

- **People who cope with their voices experience what their voices say more as statements or opinions and seldom as commands.** Why should voices not also have an opinion? Sometimes that opinion will sound like a command. If I say 'I don't like your hat' and I happen to sound like a dominating teacher at the school you attended, it may sound like I am strongly suggesting that you take the hat off. It is important that you help your client towards a more pragmatic view of things and help them to limit reading into experiences messages that may not actually be there. You will probably find that they have had to learn to read messages into what people are implying. As one of my clients once said, 'I have to try to decode what my father says.' In this case, the father had not actually 'said' anything barring a few grunts and heavy breathing, but this was against a background of an explosive personality. No wonder then that some voice-hearers who have had similar experiences are inclined to make negative appraisals about communication automatically; in their history such appraisals may have had a lot of survival value.

Ⓡ Routledge Taylor & Francis Group

- **People who cope with their voices attempt to conduct an assertive conversation with their voices and set limits as to the influence the voices have in the relationship.** The one-sidedness of the relationship with the voices has to be brought to an end. In the rampant voice-hearing experience, the voice talks and the voice-hearer listens and defers to the voice. At the very least, this is undemocratic. The voice-hearer needs to learn to throw down the gauntlet of debating with almost every issue the voice brings up, even if they are in the grip of anxiety. The voice naturally does not have to pick up this gauntlet. So when a voice-hearer tells you that the strategy you suggested here 'did not work', it is necessary to point out that the aim of the exercise is not for the voice-hearer to become a dictator; you cannot force anyone to talk if they do not want to. The aim of the exercise is really to move the voice-hearer from being passive in the relationship to a more active interactional role in which exchanges rather than bullying take place.

- **People who cope with their voices communicate fairly often about their voices.** Voice-hearers do not like talking about their voices for many reasons. A significant one often cited is that they are scared of their voices' reaction should they discuss them with someone else. It is as if they accept that Big Brother is listening. Many a voice-hearer also firmly believes that the voice can physically harm them or alternatively force them to harm themselves. This latter fear may well be valid and should be born in mind by the clinician. Only when the voice-hearer has reached a greater level of confidence in their power in the relationship can one steadily move forward on this issue. However, it should never be entirely set aside. Because we are inclined to preferentially tote up our failures or the bad things that happen, we do not notice when expected bad things do *not* happen. This is also true of voice-hearers. Thus, when they talk about their voices with no bad consequences this should be pointed out to them. This chronically happens in ward rounds where voices are often freely discussed with no known consequences. This should be pointed out to the client. Tread carefully, however; there will be many instances that your voice-hearer will point out when there apparently were bad effects.

- **People who cope with their voices commonly use focusing (non-avoidance) strategies.** The voice-hearer needs to be helped to abandon avoidance as a primary strategy. Because this is so important, I will explain the difference between avoidance and focusing strategies later.

I feel so strongly about avoidance as a strategy that I would like to expand on it. Although retired, I still hear about how clinicians are trying to cope with people who hear voices. It seems like many a clinician still advocates avoidance. For example, one of the most popular techniques on offer is 'Turn the radio on'.

Routledge
Taylor & Francis Group

That avoidance is advocated was also the case while I was still in practice. Given the outcomes of the mini-projects with training clinicians, it is worth speculating on the reasons for this.

> **Avoidance is a short-term strategy that keeps anxiety high and offers no lasting effect.**

You may not be aware of it but when anyone uses avoidance strategies, they are exposing themselves to operant conditioning.[1] Operant conditioning plays a role in all addictions from gambling through to substance abuse. It is so powerful because it rewards on a random basis.

> **Avoidance strategies contain powerful conditioning elements through which your voice-hearer may become addicted to avoidance.**

Working with people who hear voices pushes a clinician into a very uncomfortable space. The phenomenon of voice-hearing does not sit easily with the Western mind. Even in ages past, people who heard voices either became the shaman or were burned at the stake. As Westerners, we just do not know where to place voice-hearing and, as such, we do not know how to relate to someone who claims to be hearing voices.

This posture has kept clinicians at a distance from working at any depth with people who hear voices. The difficulty is, however, that eventually clinicians have to get to grips at the pit face, but they do not know how or where to start. Naturally, there is the readily available medication, which I believe relieves the stress as much for the clinician as it does work to sedate the client. This is not a healthy state of affairs for either the clinician or the voice-hearer as both are trapped in a management regimen. Both groups know that the problem will return. Both will again feel the same discomfort. Both will again only have one strategy to use.

I hope I can share here some of the practical techniques I have used to deal with my own and similar dilemmas as well as those of voice-hearers with clinicians. I did not develop these techniques. It is just a matter of seeing and using them in an integrated fashion.

The techniques are not new; they are actually staring us all in the face and there is a good evidence base for using these tools. Some of the big names in developing them are Marius Romme and Sandra Escher and all of the authors who dealt with the power dynamics in relationships, such as Jay Haley and his tutors. Then there are the cognitive behavioural people

Routledge
Taylor & Francis Group

who focused on psychosis, including Richard Bentall, Phillipa Garety, Max Birchwood, Paul Chadwick, Tony Morison and many others. Among this esteemed gathering I would like to mention Irvin Yalom, the master of group therapy, as he focused on and highlighted the power of relationship dynamics.

At the core of applying the techniques the clinician has to identify that working with troublesome voices is largely about dealing with a person's interpretation of an experience and their response to that interpretation. As a clinician you will be directing your energies towards changing the process (interpretations, meanings and actions of the client) from something that is ultimately self-defeating[2] and malignant, to something that is benign. The self-defeating earlier process is moved towards a process that assists the voice-hearer to resume a fulfilling life.

> *Your central area of work lies within the voice-hearer's interpretation of experiences and how they translate this into behaviour.*
>
> *Ultimately, behaviour should work for rather than against the person.*

You can never promise the person that their voices will be removed but you can offer them the opportunity to change the kind of relationship they have with their voices from one of subordination, deference and fear to one of parity. In this sense it is no different from what we all desire and – it is hoped – actively strive for in our various relationships: equality.

3.2 Your orientation and attitude

Perhaps before embarking headlong and striking out into the great unknown of strategic work with a person who hears voices, you – the clinician – also need to have a look at where you stand with regard to voices and voice-hearers.

- If you believe that people who hear voices cannot change, it will show. You need to review where you stand on this issue.

- If you believe that your client is shamming, manipulating or seeking attention, you are starting off on the wrong foot. Reserve your judgement; you will soon learn that none of the above applies to the voice-hearing experience. I will expand on this further at the end of this list.

- The statement 'The client is also an expert' needs to be considered seriously. Does the client know anything that you don't? Think about it.

- Are you prepared to be creative? For example, make use of drawings and other representations (that may be metaphors) to help your client understand something you are trying to get across and also that you are trying to understand their thinking style.

- It is always useful to have as many skills at your disposal as possible. Are you prepared to buff-up your breadth of clinical skills? Try to see how they overlap and how you can use key concepts to help you understand your client.

- Do you think you could assume a student role? You need to be open to your client 'teaching' you about their frame of reference.

- Beware of your own model of practice, core training and personal beliefs. You may have very strong views about how certain things work; you may feel defensive about adding to or letting go of some of these beliefs. Do not be afraid of change in yourself and in your practice.

- Are you prepared to try to absorb new ideas from your client and others? If, for some or other reason, you believe that you are not allowed to change, you are limiting yourself and thus you are limiting your therapeutic frame of reference. This means that your client could be losing out on something that could be very helpful.

- You will need to become client-centred and collaborative.

This means:

- Also use the material the client brings. Work with their ideas, thoughts and feelings.

- Only introduce material that they can understand and cope with at that moment. Anyone's ability to concentrate waxes and wanes throughout the day. Never force anything beyond the person's ability at that time. Be sensitive to the person's 'state' at the time that you want to introduce something.

- Family or carer involvement must fit into your treatment plan: it is not uncommon that the person's distress often occurs within a certain context. Family and friends play a big role in the person's life. Carers sometimes accidentally maintain the person's self-defeating responses to their voices. There is not a lot of sense to go on trying to help the person in isolation when, as soon as they get back into their usual environment, all of your efforts are blown away.

- Intervene early. Act on your suspicion of deterioration in the client. What are you waiting for – a breakdown? Work preventively. You need to investigate the use of relapse prevention

Routledge
Taylor & Francis Group

(see Appendix 10). This will generate a relapse signature that you and the client will find useful. Having a relapse signature places at least part of the power for recovery in the person's hands.

- Maintain contact. Your client finds working with their voices unpleasant; this unpleasantness is sometimes worse than the unpleasantness of living with voices. With this conflict in place, your client may actively work towards sabotaging their contact with you. This is quite common. They want to be left alone. It is not an option to let them stew with their voices; the longer the process goes on without break, the more it will embed. Voices have to be continuously harassed out of existence. Never give up.

> ***Working with voice-hearers requires that you examine where you stand on a variety of issues.***

I would now like to return to the rather unproductive thought we all have and that will enter your mind when you meet any voice-hearer. It is the question about whether this client is trying to seek attention or is manipulating you for some kind of gain. Although there are some people who may do that, I have never found that to be the case with people who experience voices. It is very difficult for a person to fake hearing voices.

- Voices as described by the voice-hearer have internal consistency. In other words, there is little if any variation of the experience over time. The 'personality' of any individual voice remains constant. This is where the phoney voice-hearer falls down badly.

- The voice-hearer experiencing voices may well show autonomic physical responses, for example, startled reactions, sweating or a dry mouth, which could not be faked.

- The process history[3] that voice-hearers provide is consistent; dates, times and circumstance are all constant over time and irrespective of who is asking the questions.

- Most of the symptoms of anxiety are commonly present. This is difficult for a pretender to fake.

- Voice-hearers do not easily talk about their voices let alone try to hop on the stage. Their reluctance is effectively diagnostic. Further, if you can get them to talk about their voices then they will continually try to move away from the topic. They will also show varying degrees of anxiety throughout the conversation. In a voice-hearers' group that I ran with other clinicians over a six-year period voice-hearers elected to have a break in the middle of the group sessions, specifically in order to de-stress.

- The voice-hearer may describe their voice-hearing experiences in complex metaphor and this also is always consistent. It may only be relaxed when the voice-hearer sufficiently trusts you. If metaphor is used it will be up to you to try to understand or unravel it. Do not write it off as some kind of disorientation or necessarily as having diminished mental capacity.[4] The metaphor will have some personal meaning for the voice-hearer. My take on why it appears is because the voice-hearer is trapped in the kind of paradox[5] that we all fall into from time to time: there is something you want to say, yet you fear the consequences of saying it. Subsequently, you produce a padded version. Sometimes the padding becomes so thick as to obscure the message.

- Looked at whichever way you like, there is nothing to be gained by having a voice. If there is any reason to have a voice it was described by Jay Haley (1963, p15): 'The crucial aspect of a symptom is the advantage it gives the patient in gaining control of what is to happen in a relationship with someone else. A symptom may represent considerable distress to the patient subjectively, but such distress is preferred by some people to living in an unpredictable world of social relationships over which they have no control.' Should this be the reason, it is an indictment of society and something we should best pay attention to in the bigger picture.

- I have found it necessary to believe what my voice-hearing clients have told me about actions they have considered when they are really distressed. Again, there may be some clients on your caseload that will try to scare you in order to get a reaction or more hospital time. Under these conditions you may be inclined to indulge in some positive risk taking without changing the way you monitor the situation. I have found that bad things can be triggered very quickly with a voice-hearer. Things that you or I may regard as insignificant may be huge for the voice-hearing person. Positive risk taking here is very risky for both client and clinician.

When you work with voice-hearers you should be aware that their experiences – past and present – place them at considerable risk.

Being entangled with a voice-hearing experience is hugely distracting. In itself, this makes voice-hearers vulnerable. However, perhaps of more concern is the danger they are to themselves. This can range from self-neglect, through social isolation (that contributes to a drop off in social skills as well as being trapped with their voices) to impulsive self-harm and frank suicide attempt. The latter may take place as a result of commands by the voices or merely because the voice-hearer has reached a tipping point as regards having voices. The action, as the tipping point is reached, could take place very impulsively. This is not the person seeking to be on stage and clinicians

Routledge
Taylor & Francis Group

would be wise to take evidence of recurring thoughts of taking one's own life (suicidal ideation) in a voice-hearer very seriously.

> **Voice-hearers are seldom attention seeking. It is best to act on risky warning signs.**

Voice-hearers are also prone to run foul of society's rules as confusion impacts on their memory and social awareness. This could result in them getting into conflicts with neighbours and possibly even the police. It is always helpful to try to limit these traumatic experiences by being mindful of what your voice-hearing clients are doing. They are not actively trying to cause trouble; their behaviour is badly misunderstood and therefore misinterpreted by John and Joan Citizen. The voice-hearer's behaviour could well be a reaction to the mere presence of voices or suggestions and commands given by their voices. On the other hand, John and Joan Citizen also have a right to a relatively trouble-free life and cannot always make space for others' behaviour even if this is due to hearing voices.

Occasionally, a voice-hearer may react to commands from their voices that could endanger the public. You need to be acutely aware of the dangers your voice-hearer, in their relationship with their voices, may pose to the public. Thus, you also have a responsibility towards the public. Monitoring, assessment and reassessment of what the voices are doing is essential. If you feel that – for whatever reason – your view of risk is clouded, you could consider requesting another clinician to have an interview with your voice-hearer. As a last resort to assess risk, you can organise a medico-legal risk assessment (a Mental Health Act Assessment in the UK).

Apart from this more formal and direct approach, you can think of some generic education of the public services in your area like the police, teachers, probation officers and alcohol and drug services. Carers' groups would also welcome your input.

> **It is helpful when those who work with voice-hearers develop an understanding of the experiences that voices-hearers have.**

Routledge
Taylor & Francis Group

3.3 Practical stuff

When people move into a new house most of them would clean it; cobwebs, dust and unidentified bits lying about will all be removed. They will try as much as they are able to start on a 'clean slate'.

Before getting into the down-to-earth practical stuff as regards dealing with voices, you also have to 'clean the slate'. Stuff that does not work, dogma and all the extraneous but impracticable and useless stuff we all have accumulated during our training and over our careers needs to go.

> *You will need to be prepared to view a voice-hearer and the idea of voice-hearing in a way that is free from dogma.*

The first of these changes is to move right away from seeing avoidance as a viable strategy. It has no long-term value while at the same time having an addictive quality and tending to keep anxiety at a high level.

Almost without exception, all my voice-hearing clients reflected that once the music from the player or TV stops, any combination of the following can happen:

- **The voices got louder.** Perhaps they meant that their voices *sounded* louder, which stands to reason if their voices were there all the time behind the noise of the music or television. The point here is that the voice-hearer *interprets* the experience as 'louder'. Louder means stronger, more powerful and more difficult to interrupt. Thus, in a perverse way suggesting avoidance may have the result of adding evidence to the belief that the voices are very powerful; it says that there is nothing you can do about your voices except blot them out with sound. The sad truth about this is that often voices can 'out-shout' any sound that the client pumps into their ears.

- **The voices were more abusive.** Do they mean that the music calmed them down and that it was a shocking experience to move from this calmer state to the startled state when the music was switched off? The point is that we don't know what the effect of music is. But what I would say is that it could not be seen as a solution but as a palliative, at best.

- **The voices stayed longer.** It is tricky to formulate this one, but the point here is that should this happen, whatever the cause, the client could view this as another threat from the voice.

Routledge
Taylor & Francis Group

This adds to the already large body of information the client has about the power of the voices. Some clients see their voices as punishing them and acutely fear this punishment. By voices staying longer, it could be seen as a punishment and may further entrench the voice-hearer's underlying belief that they are powerless.

- **The voices were gone but then I worried about when they would come back.**
  This is completely understandable because the voices have played this trick before. Voice-hearers often feel tricked or trapped or caught out by their voices. Thus, staying away and then arriving unannounced is just another one of the nasty tricks that voices produce. It has also occurred to some voice-hearers that this game-playing quality of voices proves that the voices win even when they are not there. What a display of power. The problem here is that this on–off process may well also perpetuate the startle response and thus the 'power' of the voices as well as keeping the voice-hearer at a higher than normal level of anxiety.

> *Stopping avoidance strategies may have the effect of the voices becoming apparently worse in some way. Avoidance strategies need to be replaced by something.*

The opposite of avoidance, that is, focusing, is well-known by clinicians. It is extensively used when treating phobias. The phobic person is encouraged to face their problem, grasp the nettle and, as it were, walk into the problem rather than turning their backs on it as if it was not there. It is therefore baffling that many a clinician still suggests avoidance strategies as the only psychological strategy to voice-hearers.

I therefore need to reiterate a rule I gave to the voice-hearers in their section:

> *Avoiding a problem does not solve it.*

Here is another:

> *Offering a strategy that suggests your client should put their head in the sand will cause them to get their butts kicked.*

In fairness, 'focusing' is a term that may be foreign to some clinicians and consequently when desensitising a phobic reaction they may not have realised that in these cases they were using focusing processes. Thus, when thinking about strategies for people who hear voices, clinicians may not have thought of focusing. Focusing is a cognitive strategy and will be discussed in more detail later.

For the moment, and in summary of all of the above, you need to accept:

> - *The voice-hearer is not seeking attention or trying to get some gain by saying that they hear voices.*
> - *What the voice-hearer is experiencing is horrifyingly real for them.*
> - *It is extremely frightening and threatening for them.*
> - *Hearing voices causes enormous anxiety in most.*
> - *If their experience is trivialised it places the voice-hearer and quite possibly others at risk.*
> - *It would be useful to get a working knowledge of a variety of approaches.*

To kick off the practical stuff, here I briefly revisit the therapeutic framework from which you will draw: a client-centred and collaborative framework; a cognitive-behavioural framework; an interpersonal-relationship framework; a systems approach; a narrative approach; the compassionate mind approach; and mindfulness. This may sound daunting, as if you have to obtain a degree in each. This is not so. Although you may not know it, you may have received informal training in several of these already. I would like to present some elements from these that I found useful when working with voice-hearers.

A client-centred and collaborative framework

This perspective means that you are listening and trying to understand where the client is coming from – how they see and experience things – rather than imposing your own interpretation on the client. You accept that although at times confused about their experiences, at the core they know what is going on. Informed choice rather than a prescribed treatment is the order of the day. Client-centredness is difficult to explain to a client and rather than a formal therapy it provides you with the vehicle within which all other approaches take place. Client-centredness brings the client into the picture: the aims that you hope to achieve are transparent. Further, although not wishing to dishearten them, they need to know that the endeavour is not a magical 'cure' for voice-hearing experiences. You will appreciate that they may well find this disappointing. However, your aim is to help them regain a life in spite of the voices and you should stress this. Illustrate this with examples of how people get to work around their difficulties and carry on with their lives in spite of their difficulties; if they can do it then so can your client.

Routledge
Taylor & Francis Group

The client's resources and experience of the situation are used and developed; the client definitely is an expert. They know what it is like to hear voices and it is these areas that require your attention. Self-defeating strategies are identified and modified so as to become more productive. Once identified, the search for alternative strategies is pursued with your client. In this respect you may suggest strategies found useful by others as well as examples from research you may have read on the topic. It still remains the client's choice if they would like to try those particular strategies.

Is client-centredness colluding? Strangely enough many clinicians have raised this question as regards client-centredness. *The Oxford Dictionary* (1982, p117) defines collusion as 'an agreement between two or more people for deceitful or fraudulent purpose'. Accepting that the client's experience is valid for them is not collusion because their experience is not necessarily valid for you. Thus, you are not endorsing the client's experience as 'reality'. You are merely trying to understand the client's experience and unravel the thought pathway they used to get to that point. As you are neither hearing voices, nor agreeing that voices may be present, this cannot easily be seen as collusion.

A cognitive, cognitive-behavioural and behavioural framework

Weaving a cognitive-behavioural thread into the process will require that you investigate what thoughts the client has and how they are acting on those thoughts. This will include what exactly the voices are saying and what they are commanding the client to do. It will also touch on personal meaning that the client attaches to all of these experiences and the effect that this has on them. In this process you will also be addressing what the client does with so-called anomalous experiences. We all have these experiences on a daily basis. They are sensory experiences that we cannot easily identify. Under conditions of high anxiety we are all inclined to assign a meaning or definition that is self-defeating to these. When this happens it is possible that self-defeating beliefs are generated about this experience. Should the perception involved be auditory, it is quite possible that it would be described in terms of a voice that then is granted certain characteristics. These tend to fit the person's unassertive momentary or generic personal and interpersonal status. Cognitive and cognitive behavioural strategies are well suited to tackle this type of problem. A parallel process often takes place when the client attempts to deal with cause. It is not unlikely that an inaccurate cause could be attached to the experience. This process is often referred to as misattribution.

Misattribution is therefore another target. The client is helped to change these attributions and consequently their reaction to them.

A cognitive-behavioural approach also includes the very important processes of reframing, dealing with confirmation bias[6] and cognitive dissonance.[7]

Reframing (Watzlawick *et al.*, 1974) actually rests on a very common process: recognising that the same thing can be seen, described and defined in different ways.

I like explaining reframing in terms of a paper clip. Waving a paper clip in the air, at training sessions I asked people to tell me what it is I was holding. After the laughter subsided I asked them at what stage would it cease to be a paper clip should I start straightening it? In other words, when would you call it something else? Further, what is it really? The name I give something defines my relationship with it. If I call it a paper clip, it is likely that I will not see its other possibilities.

> *Being blind to something's possibilities limits flexibility and adaptability.*

Similarly, if I have named a relationship as hostile it will be difficult to shift from that position. Strangely, I will actively look for elements of hostility in that or similar situations. This is a normal process and is known as a confirmation bias. Should I find the smallest piece of evidence, logical or not, it will confirm my hypothesis. In turn, this will influence my behaviour within that or similar situations. Reframing rests on the fact that when I name something, that name comes with a package of qualities to which I then respond in a fairly stereotyped way.

Reframing therefore facilitates a perceptual shift between

- objects (it is not necessarily a person in your room; it could be a shadow)
- functions (your voice may not be targeting you; it may just be frustrated with you)
- inherent qualities (the voice is not bad; it just has a gruff way of saying things).

There will also be various combinations of the above.

It is also important to note some key functional qualities of reframing:

- Although unusual, each alternative description of the object or experience must be valid, possible and realistic.
- Take care not to present a person with a view that is too different from their currently held

Routledge Taylor & Francis Group

views as this could result in rejection of the message. In this process you, as the sender of the message, may also be discredited to an extent.

- Use any strategy sparingly. Each strategy you apply is part of a bigger strategic process. Because of its nature, repeatedly applying reframing may make you seem domineering and always having to have the last word, which is also a quality of voices.

- Reframing is meant to trigger cognitive dissonance – certainly not to persuade the person that your interpretation is the 'right' one.

Cognitive dissonance was first described in Festinger's *A Theory of Cognitive Dissonance* (1957). The theory was never fully embraced, yet is an exceptionally powerful tool in the store of cognitive-behavioural techniques. As such, voice-hearers can benefit from its use, in which a dysfunctional belief about the attributes – for example, the power – of the voices is tackled. Its aim is to weaken this position of power that the client has granted to it.

Purely as an example of how cognitive dissonance could be employed with voice-hearers: we all make mistakes in our communications, no less voices, and you can utilise the mistakes that voices make. They often communicate in vague or metaphorical terms that can be wedged apart by highlighting contradictions in how they behave. Discrepancies, inaccuracies and apparent reasoning errors in what the voice is saying are pointed out to the client. The client is now left to deal with these discrepancies in their voice's communication that will cause cognitive dissonance for them.

Cognitive dissonance is never forced home; the client is left to sort out the dissonance themselves, unless they want to speak about it. You may never see the actual workings of cognitive dissonance; however, you may notice a shift in your client's attitude and behaviour toward the voices. See Table 2 for illustrations of cognitive dissonance.

 Routledge Taylor & Francis Group

Table 2: Illustrations of cognitive dissonance

Cognition = Belief	Cognition = Perception
I support political party XYZ because of their honesty.	Several senior members are involved in financial scams.
Aggression is unacceptable.	I often lose my temper badly.
My voices are all-powerful.	My voices respond to some of my requests and instructions.

It is important that the dissonant statement that you introduce should not be shocking to the person. If this happens, it is easy for the person to reject the dissonant statement. Strategies aimed at changing a belief or attitude cannot be expected to be effective through the application of a one-off event. Thus, although you may never actually enquire as to whether the cognitive dissonance worked, should your client bring up the subject that triggered your use of it, you can then reapply it. I would, however, suggest that you do so from a slightly different perspective. In other words, do not repeat your strategy verbatim.

Clinical example of cognitive dissonance

In a group therapy session for voice-hearers, a client told us that she had bought a new toaster but no sooner had she brought the item home when one of her voices suggested that she should electrocute herself with it. She never even opened the box. After some thought we put it to her that as it was clear that at times she misunderstands verbal communication from people, could it also be that she may at times misunderstand what her voices are saying to her? Somewhat reluctantly she agreed. We then went on to suggest that perhaps the voice had said, 'You could (rather than "should") electrocute yourself.' The two communications now fall into different classes. The initial one was a command (dominant, controlling) whereas the one we suggested was a health warning (friendly, not controlling). This then has implications for how she defines the voice. In her first interpretation she is confirming that the voice commands and is allowed to command her, thus verifying her subordinate position. In the second instance, the voice is at worst neutral and at best a 'good' voice. The cognitive dissonance lies therein that she is now left with the possibility of seeing the voice in a different light. The two opposing views – 'the voice is powerful' and 'the voice may be helpful sometimes' – have to be resolved by the person. The client did eventually get to use the toaster, without further prompting or

---

Routledge Taylor & Francis Group

reference from us. The seeds of doubt are left for the client to resolve. Can you see that reframing is also used in this case? Reframing often causes a cognitive dissonance; the two often go together.

A similar example was provided by Romme and Escher at the Psychosis International Conference in Perth (5 November 2008). A client, Ami, reported: 'My relationship with my voices changed when I learned to see them as a signal of my problems and I learned to react positive to them. When they said to me, "Look at her – what a disaster," I looked in the mirror and thought they are right – I should dress more properly.' From a negative influence it became a stimulus. Ami had flipped what the voices were saying on its head. This is the reframing move that caused the dissonance. She now had two opposing views of what the voice was actually saying. She did this by listening to what they were saying, avoiding her common knee-jerk interpretation that it was bad and rather looking for a useful message in it. Her point of departure was that perhaps the voices were trying to tell her something useful; all she had to do was to decode it.

Challenging beliefs about voices

There are many beliefs that in particular support the power of voices. Some of the typical ones that I have heard are:

- If I question my voices then something bad will happen to me.
- My voices get louder at night.
- My voices can harm me.
- My voices are other people's thoughts being forced into my head.

Voice-hearers seem to be eternally negative about their resilience on the one hand and the power of their voices to overwhelm them on the other. Well, for them this is true; they have plenty of evidence that they will place before you. The trick is finding the flaw in the evidence. Here, too, cognitive dissonance will again be useful with statements by you such as, 'Isn't it just possible that …?' or 'You know, another one of my clients had a similar experience,' and then, without revealing any personal details, you go on with, 'They found that if they did (X), then (A) and (B) and (C) were the outcomes.'

As a matter of interest, this strategy actually also incorporates what Yalom (1975) sees as a curative factor and calls 'universality' in group therapy. It lets the person know that their experience is similar to another person's. Thus, it simultaneously tackles the isolation of the voice-hearer with their voices.

Ⓡ Routledge
Taylor & Francis Group

There are many more. These pessimistic beliefs add to the voice-hearer's feelings of being powerless and/or perpetuate the apparent power of the voice. In a measured way, these beliefs need to be challenged and eroded.

Focusing versus avoidance

Focusing means guiding the person towards, and helping them to look at, the problem, in spite of the anxiety that doing such produces. It literally focuses on the feared object and handling it. Focusing is grasping the nettle. It is while focusing on the feared object or thought that solutions are found. There is nothing mystical about this. If I am using a circular saw, it is best that I look at it even if I see it as dangerous and scary. Naturally, this process, like all desensitisation[8] processes, takes place in a graded way. Bear in mind that what you are doing is stressful for the client; you are asking them to tackle a frightening, abusive and very powerful adversary. It is for this reason that you walk softly and have patience.

Focusing gives the person the opportunity to study the problem and then to explore ways of addressing it because, after having studied the problem, the person is better placed to exploit the weak points of the problem. By knowing the dimensions of the problem, the client is better placed to make choices about how to deal with it.

Sun Tzu (*c.* 500 BC) pointed out that if you know your enemy and you know yourself then 'you will never be defeated … in a hundred battles'.

Thus, focusing and avoidance contain some stark differences; whereas focusing is a forward-moving, hands-on approach, avoidance backs off, and does not seek a solution to the problem. Avoidance also contains elements of panic. Panic, in turn, is in phase with anxiety, if not part of it. Anxiety, as we know, cannot be used profitably in problem solving. Nothing fundamental can be expected to change when avoidance is used.

Typical processes present in focusing strategies are:

- facing a problem by recognising its existence
- analyzing the problem by trying to unravel it
- using problem-solving techniques such as those that are used in behavioural family therapy, which I have adapted from Fadden *et al* (2012):

R Routledge
Taylor & Francis Group

1 Identify the target problem.
2 Between you and the voice-hearer think of as many solutions as possible. Write them down, including the ones that seem hopeless or ineffectual at first glance; they could always be modified to be more effective later.
3 Choose the 'best' one, keeping the others in reserve.
4 Bear in mind that there often are no 'best' ones.
5 Practice it several times.
6 Hone it to work better.
7 Accept that no single strategy 'does it all'.

Focusing means assisting the voice-hearer to:

- take a risk to tackle the voices; if it is too scary then they can always – temporarily and strategically – retreat, knowing that they will eventually come back
- recognise and understand the patterns of the voices and their response to them (When do they come? What do I do then? Does my response work in the longer term?)
- deal with the problem, not with something or someone else; displacement activity[9] should be limited, or, better still, replaced with focusing techniques
- reflect on achievements
- be creative in formulating portable strategies themselves; dependence on you (even for prompting) for strategies is a contra-indicator to change. (Look back at the voice-hearer I met at the London conference mentioned in Chapter 1.)

Focusing is looking into the face of the problem and doing something about it, however small or illogical it may seem at the time.

Focusing strategies will therefore always involve some or other active, open, hands-on work with the voices, aspects of them and how the voice-hearer responds to them.

There are many ways of doing this but I would like to single out one that is of paramount importance, that of the voice-hearer trying to form a dialogue[10] with his or her voices.

Dialogue involves starting a conversation or having an exchange of ideas.
Dialogue is more than just a single word.

Routledge Taylor & Francis Group

The reason I lay such emphasis on dialogue is that it seems to target several areas of negativity in the voice-hearing experience at the same time. The most important of these I believe is that the person starts learning and practising assertiveness techniques; they move from an interactionally passive position to an interactionally active position.

Dialogue with voices is the crux of the approach that Romme (1998) derived from his work with Patsy Hage. However, it is one of the things that clinicians, voice-hearers and carers find difficult to swallow because to most people it seems very strange to have a conversation with voices. Many voice-hearers have said to me that people will think they are mad if they are seen doing this. Perhaps this is true, but every day in town and even in my own home I see people talking to other people I cannot see or hear; they are using their mobile phones. Thus, perhaps if they feel they need to say something to their voice while they are in public, they merely have to take out their mobile phone, dial the talking clock and have a conversation with their voice. This was originally suggested by Ron Coleman[11] at one of the many talks he gave.

The fact that the voice is not visible or that they are the only one who is having the experience is actually irrelevant. What is important is to change the type of relationship that is taking place.

The voice may not reply in words. However, Watzlawick *et al* (1967, p49) reminds us: 'You cannot not communicate.' Thus, even silence says something. Once again, think here of a normal relationship; if you try starting a conversation with someone and that person does not answer, what would you do? Why do anything different with a voice (that would only give the voice special status)? The problem with a voice-hearer and a silent voice is that most voice-hearers immediately define the silence as a powerful position on the part of the voice. But, as we know, silence could mean many things.

Thus, if a voice remains silent when the voice-hearer attempts dialogue, they could comment on the silence: 'Pardon me, perhaps you did not hear me …?' Alternatively, the silence could be reframed so as to put the voice at a disadvantage and thus the voice-hearer in an advantageous position. For example, the voice-hearer could point out the weak stance by the voice when it is silent: 'You seem to be at a loss for words.' The voice-hearer could also add a sting to the last observation by adding: 'If you don't want to talk, that's OK.'

Should the voice get angry, the voice-hearer should not define this as a powerful position; the voice-hearer must be helped not to respond with either anger or fear under these conditions.

Ɍ Routledge
Taylor & Francis Group

They should remember that angry people are a bit out of control and thus off balance. They could try: 'I'm sorry you are getting angry; would you like some time to calm down?'

> *To make the point again, the voice-hearer changes their position in the relationship from passive to active, from deferential to assertive.*

The above process is very much also part and parcel of an interpersonal-relationship perspective.

An interpersonal-relationship framework

Earlier I drew attention to the view that a voice-hearer is locked into a one-sided relationship with their voices in which the voice is in the dominant position. The aim of this framework is to address the power imbalance existing in the relationship.

As a guide to understanding this framework and how to use it you need to consider that Haley (1963) suggested that there are three positions of power in a relationship and indeed within the individual transactions within a relationship. It may seem strange to bring it down to this level but the power play within the relationship with a voice works at this micro level.

In any relationship there are fluctuations between the positions of dominance the two parties hold in that relationship, even on a moment-by-moment basis. At times it is person 'A' who is holding what is known as the 'one-up' position; at times it is person 'B' who is holding that position. Thus, in a relationship there are three power slots available for one person relative to the other: one-up, equal or one down. Graphically, this can be represented as follows (see Figure 6), where the arrows indicate the dominant direction of communication:

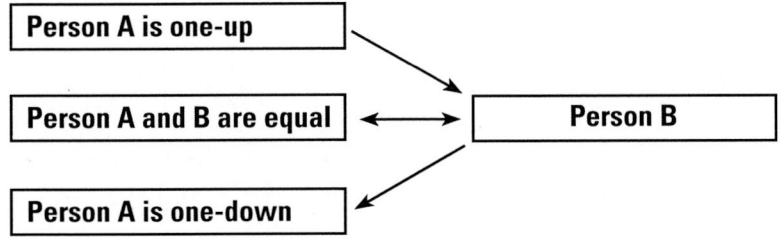

Figure 6 Power slots in a relationship

In the case of a relationship with a voice, the voice-hearer is predominantly in the one-down slot; the voice is instructing, demanding and abusing with little or no resistance from the voice-hearer.

In this respect, it is interesting that Birchwood (2006) seemed also to be alluding to there being a relationship of power between voice and voice-hearer. He indicated that the deferential way that people relate to their voices could be a reflection of their social relationships (their social rank in their group). He went on to ask what was driving the subordinate role. Was it depression? Was it the relentless nature of voices? His findings indicated that it was neither depression nor the frequency of the voice but could well have something to do with the subordinate role.

In many of our group members it was clear that the person often occupied a subordinate interpersonal position by default. This was regularly also the position occupied in the family. There were instances when this default one-down position had occurred over time in a significant relationship, or it could have developed as a result of short-lived but sharp psychological trauma, or a combination of both. Such a subordinate position is quickly adopted and may even be embedded in people in a hostage situation, for example. The term 'hostage' can be used in a broad sense and, as such, people can be held 'hostage' in many ways.

> You will remember the case I mentioned earlier of the young man whose father had a rather explosive temperament and who would, on occasion, settle himself in the lounge in the presence of his son. Father would then, for whatever reason, proceed to breathe heavily and make various grunts. This condition left the young man wondering if there was some message for him in his father's behaviour and if it heralded some explosion. Remaining in the room became like a hostage situation.

A systems approach

A systems approach is not to be confused with what is known generally as a 'systemic' approach, which commonly refers to the use of systemic family therapy. A systems approach, very broadly speaking, takes note of the fact that no one is an island. It subsumes systemic family therapy. Its principles were derived by Ludwig von Bertalanffy (1968), a mathematician who described these principles in his general system[12] theory.

When viewing any problem from a system theory perspective you need to note how various elements of the problem interact and how changes in one area will affect all the others.

Routledge
Taylor & Francis Group

This presupposes that you have an overview of those elements that are stakeholders in the person's life. Remember, too, that as soon as you engage with a system you become part of it. Consequently, you cannot ever be an observer of a system, only a participant.

> *You can never view your client objectively because you also influence them as well as those around them, and they influence you.*

Many clinicians lose sight of this fact by failing to recognise how they influence the stakeholders in the system and also how they are influenced by the various processes in the system.

You may notice these effects in yourself. For example, you probably behave differently when you are around your parents than when you are around your friends. This will again probably change in the presence of both your friends and your parents.

In a voice-hearer these system effects may show up as the activation of voices when certain people or thoughts about them are present. To get a more comprehensive understanding of my clients' dilemmas, it has in many cases been important that I meet with a voice-hearer both out of and within the family set-up. Only seeing a client out of the usual context they occupy often therefore provides a distorted picture; it certainly will provide incomplete and poor-quality information, making formulation and thus treatment less effective.

I could only get insight into some of the drivers of some clients' anxiety by seeing what happened at home. In many cases I have been astounded at the abuse that takes place; it may be low level but it is constant. Abuse of this nature can take on a vast number of forms.

> In one case, a family meeting struggled to get off the ground as the dad was holding forth about his problems. The client – who was supposed to be the focus of the meeting – was being sidelined. Although this certainly was not the intention, it was the effect. Clearly, this may have been the case at home as well and it raised the question about how much concerned listening was in fact able to take place in this family. Everyone was reduced to an audience for the dad.

This phenomenon is not meant to illustrate that the family environment is toxic; however, it is a very important environment into which the person is tied. The relationship with the peer group attains equal importance during the teen years. This certainly has to be taken into account as well but it is seldom that you will directly be able to see the types of interactions that take place here.

Thus, a systems approach does not only look at the family; it will include as well, for instance, the client's GP practice. In most cases I found GPs to be extremely helpful and cooperative; however, that could not necessarily be said for all the staff at some surgeries.

In another case, one of my clients had to be taken to a specialist medical unit after a suicide attempt. I was astounded at how dangerous – relatively speaking – the place was for a person with suicidal thoughts. For example, the staff had little or no awareness of indicators of suicide risk in people with diagnosed mental health problems. Further, there were elements close at hand that could have facilitated a suicide attempt by the client. I found it necessary to have a meeting with the senior staff and managers to express my concerns, which they took on board. It was not because the treatment was faulty; it was because this particular unit rarely got patients fresh from a suicide attempt.

Another point derived from the systems approach is that clients, particularly if they are in hospital, occupy a naturally one-down position with staff. Paradoxically, then, there exists within the relationship between worker and client the seeds of the same type of relationship that the client has with their voices.

There is little point in working on equality in one key relationship while denying it in another.

Often, therefore, bridging the system's cracks may require some education. Systems that are not functioning effectively do need to be addressed – be these systems in families, work situations, clinical teams, and/or friends.

In system processes one of the chief culprits is therefore ignorance; that is not a crime.

Do not expect everyone involved to understand your voice-hearing clients' needs, particular situation and what they may be at risk of. These matters need to be brought into the picture.

The compassionate mind approach

The compassionate mind approach directly targets the ways in which we all deal with ourselves. We are seldom aware of just how frequently we handle ourselves in a destructive way. To manage voices effectively the client needs to develop a resilient self-worth (see Appendix 1).

Routledge
Taylor & Francis Group

Belittling and continually attacking themselves, failing to recognise success and generally treating themselves as secondary to others (including voices) perpetuates the negative situation. Many times I have found it necessary to point out to my clients that they often sound like the prosecuting council, the judge, the jury and the executioner. I also linked this to the way that the voices treated them and left them to think about that.

Being compassionate to oneself does not mean being self-indulgent. At first it is a strange concept but eventually it makes an awful lot of sense. It also provides the client with more resilience in the face of abuse. For more in-depth reading on the compassionate mind approach see any of the relevant works by Paul Gilbert.

Mindfulness

Anna Solly's (2005) description of mindfulness is very useful. In this vein, mindfulness can be used to help voice-hearers; it could alter the relationship with the voices if the voice-hearer could:

- look at their own experiences objectively; liking and disliking do therefore not play a role
- accept the fact that sometimes things must progress in their own way and time; continually making demands on the voices to go may well have the opposite effect, whereas accepting that the voices are here now, but may not always be, can develop a better working relationship with them
- try to see every experience as new each time; the client does not wait for or listen for the voices and should they arise an "Oh, it's you again" attitude is striven for
- develop a kinder approach and attitude towards themselves (also part and parcel of the compassionate mind approach)
- pursue the goal of being themselves; in terms of their relationship with voices, this would mean that the client ultimately makes the choices about their own actions, in spite of the demands and threats issued by their voices
- work towards seeing things as they are here and now; if something is a given or a fact, it makes little sense wasting time and energy opposing it and, in fact, being continually embattled keeps stress and anxiety at high levels, providing voices with an open stage
- consider that the thrust and parry of the relationship with voices can become an all-consuming habit; although dealing with voices on an ongoing basis is necessary, there is also a time of stepping back to break away from the frenetic habit. Beyond the more formal therapeutic approaches, clinicians should also consider some social-behavioural strategies.

R Routledge Taylor & Francis Group

Breaking the isolation

Voice-hearers are very much inclined to isolate themselves from social contact. Withdrawal is common. This means that they are, more than ever, stuck with and vulnerable to their voices' demands and behaviour. Even if questioned, they seldom talk about their voices to anyone. It is for these reasons that proactive engagement is necessary with people who hear voices. It is not enough to get the voice-hearer into an activity with others; the point is to try to get them to talk about their voices with someone other than you. This implies that this other person (or people) needs some understanding of the voice-hearer's point of view. On the other hand, it is also important that people who help voice-hearers relate to the voice-hearer without being patronising or a pseudo-therapist. Forging these relationships has to be conducted with due care as both voice-hearer and others involved need to be safe with one another in its broader as well as a specific sense.

Pursuing a valued role

By isolating themselves, the voice-hearer fosters a reduction in or even the dropping of everyday activities. This includes not only a work or college situation but also the everyday, usual things we all do. Consequently, apart from becoming rusty in their occupational pursuits, they also become socially deskilled. Beyond these more obvious areas, common leisure activities are also effectively brought down to zero. The stimulation, relaxation and health benefits gained from these activities are also then lost. Planning for the future suffers in all these domains and they are left in a grey social limbo.

As a result of the battering they receive from their voices, they have accepted a stamp of being worthless and often see themselves as incapable of doing anything. Getting back to where they were before they heard voices is challenging. It is therefore important to assist them to regain, or, alternatively, cultivate, a valued role. This is not just related to paid employment; every one of us has some form of recreation, such as jogging or listening to music. The key element here, however, is that it should preferably imply some regular social contact. Thus, if the person's major hobby is collecting stamps then they could be encouraged to visit stamp fairs or join a local stamp-collecting society. There is a social component possible even in what may seem to be the most singular of activities.

We are group creatures. There are always opportunities for social activity.

Awareness of set-ups

A set-up[13] is not planned, neither is it engineered by anyone. Be that as it may, a set-up can often be seen to exist and/or can be seen to be forming. Set-ups are, however, most commonly seen with hindsight. The expression 'I should have seen that coming' is an illustration of this.

Set-ups with voice-hearers are common. The milieu within social isolation creates a cohort of set-ups that makes social deskilling, anxiety, stress and abuse more probable. Thus, a person may show recovery or progress but as soon as they re-enter their old life, the conditions there apply the same pressures that played a role in the development of voice-hearing in the first place. As an example in the physical sense, I often wonder why people who have had multiple injuries from participating in extreme sports and have needed operations because of this return to participating in such activities. Clearly, the sport has not changed; it contains the same dangers as before. Unless they have gained insight into how they dealt with the situation, most likely the person will probably approach these dangers in the same way that led to getting injured in the first place.

Similarly, a voice-hearer returning to any environment that is abusive and/or threatening predicts a poor outcome. Some of these environments are quite subtle — for example, leaving the family home for the first time and entering a busy, high-demand situation in which the person has to cope on their own.

In the early intervention team we found that this condition is a set-up for difficulties, whatever they may turn out to be. Leaving home for the first time and, for example, going to residential university, in many cases seemed to play a role in initial breakdown. This does not mean that there is anything inherently wrong with residential universities; it is merely a set of conditions that naturally places a collective pressure on a young, perhaps vulnerable, person. Often the person arrives at university already having a rich process history that may or may not have been visible. A clinician, after making progress with a client should, without molly-coddling their client, consider the pressures in the system to which the client is wishing to return. Also, in cases of discharge from a stay in hospital, the client could be returning to a very toxic environment.

> **Remember, a set-up is a set of conditions that favours a certain outcome.**
>
> **Events that may seem trivial for the clinician may be very difficult for the voice-hearer.**

Routledge Taylor & Francis Group

A narrative approach

Although the full range of narrative techniques are not necessarily employed, the phenomenon of hearing voices is embedded in a story. Knowledge of that story is a necessary asset in the skills inventory of the clinician as well as the voice-hearer. Of particular interest is how the story is organised in the client's mind. The client's narrative may well clarify links and understanding in the development of voice-hearing. Although this knowledge may not imply a specific strategy or strategies, it nonetheless removes the mystery, simply because we are seldom aware of our own narrative. Mystery accompanying voices gives them all the more power. Discovering the warp and weft of a client's narrative thus assists normalising the cause of difficulties; it is natural to develop unusual coping strategies or responses in unusual circumstances. War is an example; factors facilitating voice-hearing are no less unusual.

Your voice-hearing client's story starts from their earliest memories. I am not talking about a clinical history. It is a process history through the client's eyes that needs to be unravelled. A process history incorporates events that the client reports as significant, particularly traumatic events or traumatising conditions and long-term processes. Here, you need to keep your eyes wide open as many a traumatised person may not recognise traumatic circumstances in their lives. For example, one of my clients who had been consistently battered by a friend had come to accept this battering as normal. Many of my clients reported 'acceptable' traumatising. This effect is also often supported, if not triggered, by a poor self-worth ('I deserve battering').

Do not expect to get the full story out in one session or in one month. As your client remembers, new pieces of their story will emerge. Also, as they begin to feel safer with you, they may be prepared to reveal some more pieces of their story.

Alongside this history, you need to be aware of the natural developmental pressures that take place in any person's life. I liked using Erik Erikson's (in Maier, 1969) model of development. If you are working more with young people you can also consider reading up on what people like Vygotsky and Piaget had to say about social and cognitive development. These interesting approaches should, however, never trump the client's personal view of their journey.

It was only when voice-hearers told me of certain events that the genesis of their voice-hearing started making sense to me. This then allowed me to more accurately develop a formulation that could show clear targets for therapy.

R Routledge
Taylor & Francis Group

I have therefore found that gathering a process history and narrative is essential to addressing core issues in the person's life.

I have mentioned the rather strange phenomenon that I have encountered with more than one client: the apparent denial of the role of psycho-social trauma in the client's life. Highlighting what is clearly a set of traumatic events and trying to link them to the voice-hearing experience thus often fell on deaf ears. Perhaps the client is not yet ready to make the link. There are many possible reasons for this. There is the possibility that a person just may not recognise experiences as having been traumatic. As mentioned, I have seen this in several clients where, for example, many of my clients had moved through some horrific experiences as a teenager but seemed to fail to recognise them as significant factors in their lives. Under these conditions it is difficult to factor these into a discussion of process history and the picture it presents. You will thus need to be sensitive to your voice-hearer's readiness to assimilate traumatic events into their process history.

Naturally, it is also possible that the explanation I offered when placed next to the reasons the client had worked out (that aliens were communicating with him) were just too different. Put another way, he solved the cognitive dissonance created by my suggestion by falling back on his interpretation. I had introduced too much, too soon.

Thus, the emergence of the story within which the genesis of voice-hearing may be embedded will most likely come out in unconnected bits and pieces, sometimes moving forward, sometimes slipping back. For this reason, you may be inclined to shelve or discard the pieces as they appear. Do not do this. View the pieces that emerge as if they are parts of wreckage from an aircraft crash; each piece of wreckage tells part of the story. As you collect these you can from time to time try to arrange them into a more coherent pattern. Ask your voice-hearer if piece 'A' has a link to piece 'M'; try to reconstruct the history of events with the help of your voice-hearer. Do not think for one moment that your voice-hearer is obstructing you by producing their narrative in this chaotic way. Indeed, the chaos reflects the size of the trauma; like any explosion, bits will be scattered far and wide. In the confused state that voices (and the history that led up to them) produce in the voice-hearer, it is understandable that searching for and picking up the pieces of their story will be an extremely difficult task on their own.

Every piece of the voice-hearer's story is relevant – even if individually a piece of that story makes no sense.

Notes

1 Operant conditioning: here I specifically stress one of its key points: it is a conditioning process during which rewards are presented on a random basis. It is a very powerful form of conditioning. BF Skinner was one of the first to describe and research operant conditioning.

2 Self-defeating behaviour: behaviour that neutralises the intention, often repeatedly.

3 Process history: the history of not just what happened but how it happened. This includes significant events, processes and phases.

4 Mental capacity: the degree of ability a person has at any one time to understand the consequences of their choices.

5 Paradox: a condition of two immediate obligations that contradict each other. It causes conflict.

6 Confirmation bias: a process in which we tend to want to confirm our beliefs, even if we know that in doing so nothing will change. Confirmation bias works against reframing and cognitive dissonance.

7 Cognitive dissonance: a theory developed by Leon Festinger in 1957. It suggests that when there is a clash between cognitions this tension has to be resolved; something must change.

8 Desensitisation: repeated and graded exposure to something fearful (or an anxiety-provoking cognition) will tend to reduce the fear and/or anxiety.

9 Displacement activities: 'occur when an animal experiences high motivation for two or more conflicting behaviours: the resulting displacement activity is usually unrelated to the competing motivations' (Tinbergen in Ingram 2009).

10 Dialogue: a conversation and/or debate between two or more people. It is more than just a few words. It is assertive, not abusive. A voice-hearer can have a dialogue with their voices.

11 Ron Coleman: a key figure in the growth and maintenance of the Hearing Voices movement.

12 System: a system consists of several elements in a dynamic relationship with one another and the whole.

13 Set-ups: a set-up is a set of interacting conditions that favours a certain outcome.

Chapter 4

For carers and family

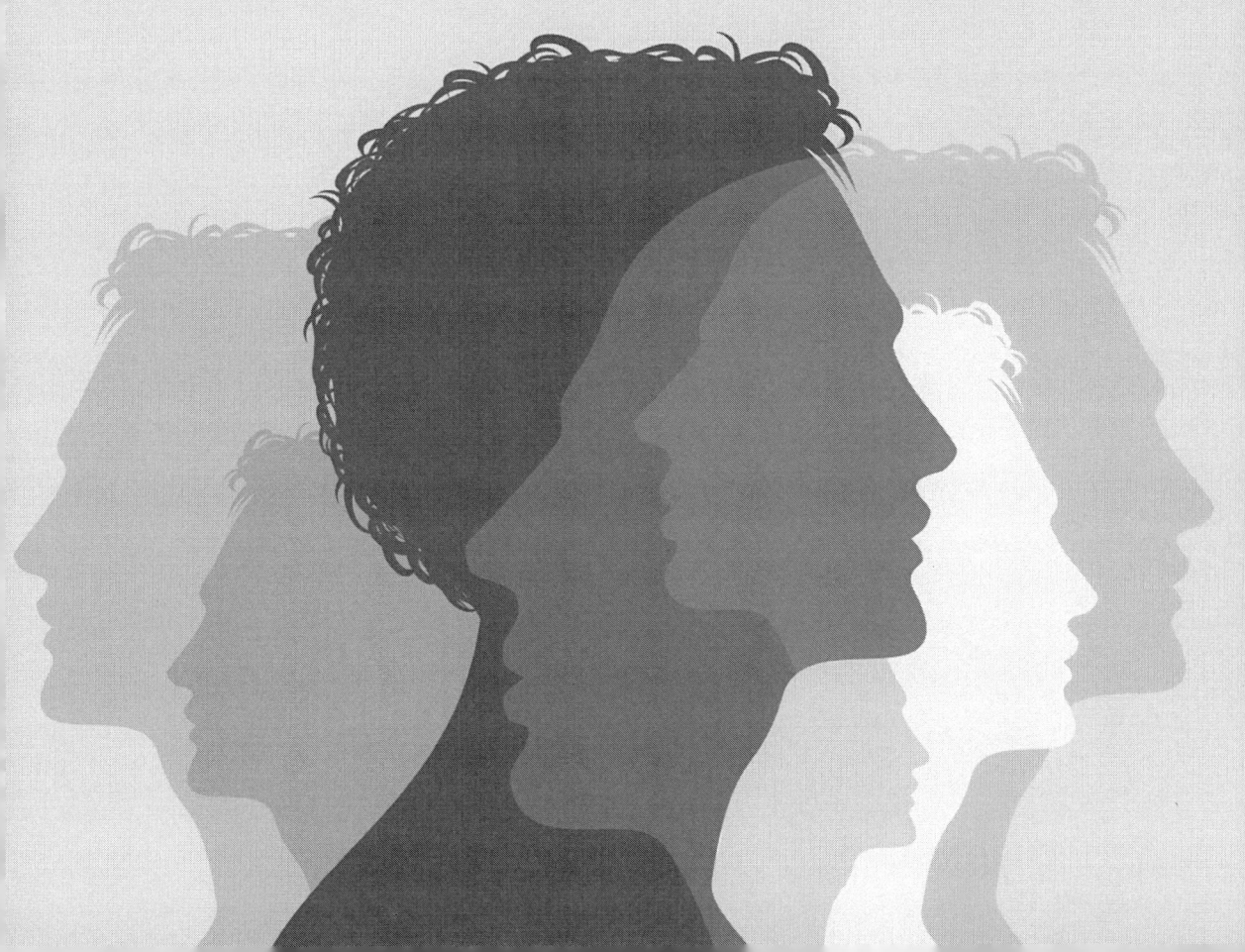

For carers and family

4.1 Loss

As a carer, you may well find this section difficult to read, but I would be lying to you if I suggested that the experience of having someone who is close to you experience domineering, abusive voices, is anything but painful. Remember, however, that I would not be writing a book of this nature if I believed there was no hope. There is hope.

> *In many cases troublesome voices can be overcome to varying degrees.*

When you learn with certainty that one of your family members has started hearing voices, it is likely that you will experience a flood of emotions. Confusion, disbelief and a sense of desperation will likely whirl around in your mind while you try to figure out this new, unknown and frightening concept. There may be the first cold touch of hopelessness as well. How do you deal with a threat, unknown and unseen? How can you consider your family member having this thing, whatever it is?

As time goes by you may slowly start tying events together. There were things that bothered you a while back but you put that down to the stress that person was going through (with the exams they were taking or with the job change or with the broken relationship or so forth). But you could never in your wildest imaginings have thought up this one: voices. What does that mean? How will they react to these 'voices'? How must I handle this person? How will I handle the situation? What will the situation be? All the questions will threaten to drown you. This process will be circular as you battle to gain understanding. It is probably the mind's way of introducing you to a new experience slowly while you struggle to understand it.

To help you understand how some parents have seen changes in their children, I have included two examples from real cases.

Example 1

Describing changes observed in a 19 year-old, Sarason (1972, p387) mentions the following:

• Changes had taken place over several months.

R Routledge
Taylor & Francis Group

- Subjects were being failed at school despite him having been a reasonable student.
- Although health conscious and good at sport, these had fallen away.
- He had withdrawn into his room and there were signs of self-neglect.

Example 2

Describing changes in her son, one mother said:

My story spans around 2 years although it feels longer, so details of events are still fresh in my mind.

My son Zak has always been a quiet, kind, placid person who managed at school and was a good skier and swimmer. At the time I did not think there was anything wrong, but, looking back, he had problems socially from adolescence.

Things went obviously wrong in 2nd year at college, when he was about 18. We put it down to a late rebellion. The kind of changes we noticed were poor attendance at school, inability to focus and mood swings. He barely managed to complete high school. Then there was a car accident that we could never get to the bottom of, when he walked home at night 4 miles in the freezing cold and bare foot. This seemed to trigger other changes. There were a series of kitchen jobs, each only lasting a few weeks at the most. He said that he was 'being poisoned' by fumes from the dishwasher or chemicals he was using.

In those early months I felt deep down that I was 'heading for a storm'; something was wrong but I didn't know what.

We thought that he perhaps needed a break and supported him on a backpack trip with friends to Central America. A week later on the trip he had a major breakdown and for a while became officially a missing person. That night became one of many 'worst nights of my life'. With the help of the High Commission he was tracked coming back the 4000 miles to the UK. He was obviously ill and referred by an insightful GP to care of mental health services.

Over the next 6 weeks he became increasingly withdrawn and hostile towards us. Sometimes he would live in the garden summerhouse, was very distressed, and in a world of his own. He was using cannabis and never touched TV, computer or music — things he used to love doing.

Source: Buckinghamshire Early Intervention Service (2007b).

Routledge
Taylor & Francis Group

In my work with families I have seen these reactions and many more. The effects on you can vary. A common effect, however, is that as the situation becomes clearer to you, your reactions fairly closely resemble bereavement. That makes all kinds of sense, as in fact you have lost someone dear to you.

Denial, clothed in the desperation of wanting to shake off this cloying, strangling reality, grips you. You want others to agree with your denial – to say it has not really happened. But really you know that it is not just a bad dream. The frustration of hopelessness and powerlessness flares up and ignites anger, sometimes reaching the level of rage. But you do not know who to blame, who to attack. You may even lash out at people close to you and those trying to help.

You feel cheated; you have put so much into bringing up this child and nurturing this relationship

You try to carry on as normal and you expect and may even insist that others also carry on as if nothing has happened. It is all part of denial.

You cannot deal with your emotions, so you force them as far away and as deep as possible until you feel emotionally numb. However, slowly pieces of the painful reality start to settle. You begin saying to yourself that your son or daughter is ill and that they will get better; it just needs time.

A candle of hope appears from somewhere; you briefly recognise the 'old' person. You wait for the improvement. As time moves on and nothing seems to be changing; you become frustrated and angry again. You start searching for the magical cure on the internet. Your GP starts taking a lot of flak from you. You want the 'right' medicine from him or her. You do not know this but probably your GP is also at a loss.

> *Being made aware that someone close to you is hearing voices may cause a reaction that looks a lot like grief.*

Routledge Taylor & Francis Group

4.2 What you will be facing

A person hearing voices may often show a variety of other symptoms, or vice versa. I do not necessarily want to go into great detail because each person displays a different set of behaviours. Suffice it to say that the person is going through their own kind of hell and you will most likely see that being expressed.

Over time and due to a variety of pressures stretching from the biological through the social and into the psychological, there has been a shift in the way they see themselves, you and the world.

The person will be in a maelstrom of anxiety and many other feelings. Thoughts only breed confusion and their world starts assuming a nightmarish proportion. Nothing stands still, and very little can be trusted. Moments of rational thought are soon wiped away as the person struggles to halt the rush in their head and get a grip on what is happening.

They may try to describe the kind of sense they are making of their own experiences but it is unlikely that what they say will make any sense to you. It could be disjointed. It could be metaphoric. It may contradict the reality you know. The anxiety that is rushing through them can cause their emotions to be extremely changeable.

As the person could be expecting some form of attack, they may become defensive, secretive, abusively hostile and perhaps even aggressive in order to protect themselves from the threats that are invading his or her mind. In extreme cases this may result in the person being admitted to hospital.

As indicated earlier, other symptoms may also precede the clear presence of voices. Whatever the case, it is important that you can recognise the phenomena when they occur.

If, unexpectedly, a person tells you that they are 'hearing voices', this may or may not be true. It depends a lot on the person's personality and your relationship with them; for example, is it a relationship of confidence and trust?

- People who hear voices may exhibit substantial reluctance in offering any information to anyone about themselves. They also do not like talking about voices because they start to feel extremely uncomfortable and anxious. There is huge fear of the response of their voices if they 'grass them up'. Further, telling people that they are hearing voices could mean they are 'mad'.

Ⓡ Routledge
Taylor & Francis Group

- People who hear voices may be difficult to engage on any topic, even those topics that used to interest them.

- People who hear voices may be socially withdrawn generally. This will really stick out if the person had previously been quite a socially active individual. This type of withdrawal is quite inflexible and may eventually result in their friends dropping them, thereby isolating them further. They will rarely seek attention and certainly will not try to use their condition to manipulate you for attention or for any gain.

- People who hear voices may abuse alcohol and/or drugs. This may be new behaviour. It is often a way of attempting to deal with voices. Naturally, this method does not work. It may in fact make the voices worse.

- People who hear voices may self-harm as a way of dealing with the voices. Naturally, this does not work and can become very risky.

Specifically, as a result of hearing voices, the following may also become apparent:

- The person appears to be reacting to something that only they are experiencing and often this happens 'out of the blue'. It may come across as distractibility. On the other hand, you may find them paying unusual and prolonged attention to the TV, particularly when people are shown talking on it.

- They will commonly appear anxious and even agitated.

- In some cases the person may ask that the TV be turned down, when in fact it is not on.

- The experiences the person has are global; they go with the person wherever they are. It would be very strange for them to hear voices in one location only; however, the voices can be triggered by common situations that may make it seem as if they are only being experienced, for instance, at home.

- Commonly, when voices turn on, the person will be startled by them. They may thus show a startle reaction. This may come across as a brief loss of concentration to what is going on around them, or they may look away, focusing at some point in the room or outside. All in all, they may come across as quite distracted and panicky.

- Voices cause distress and often disable the person socially, and thus everyday common tasks, such as getting up in the morning, attending to personal hygiene and other personal responsibilities like paying bills may be 'neglected'.

Ⓡ Routledge
Taylor & Francis Group

In order to move towards what you can do and what you should try to avoid I want to reiterate the way I approach the problem of voice-hearing.

The methods I use were profoundly influenced by my direct work with voice-hearers. Due to this, the following became apparent to me:

- The person's behaviour indicates that they are communicating with something.

- The person is in a complex relationship with that something.

- The person is subordinate to that something; it is intimidating them.

- The person is commanded, instructed, shouted at, cursed at and degraded by that something.

- The person is distressed and this often escalates. This may happen for no reason that is clear to you.

- During this distress, the person is sensitive, anxious and emotionally unpredictable.

- The person tries to deal with this something chiefly by attempting to avoid and/or exclude that something from consciousness. This may include substance abuse to dumb the experience down.

- The strategies that the person employs have little or no lasting effect, or may even make the situation worse.

- The person keeps employing these same strategies although they have no lasting effect.

- All of the above grants the person no gain in any way whatsoever. It is certainly not a case of attention seeking.

The person you knew may be very different from the one who is now hearing troublesome voices.

Because of this:

- You may find that your advice is unwelcome and may make the situation worse. This is because it may be interpreted as a demand, particularly if you are the parent. This does not preclude you from trying to help. Do not take offence; you are dealing with someone who is hyper-sensitive to anything that places demands on them.

Routledge
Taylor & Francis Group

- Talking to your voice-hearer, particularly if there are communications in which you continually draw attention to *your* distress or expectations, will just be adding another 'voice' to the voices already being heard. However, this does not prevent you from talking about your own feelings. They should be expressed in the first person, using 'I feel …' rather than 'You make me feel …' or 'It makes me feel …'. Try to strike a balance between your situation and theirs.

- Instructions, remonstrating, scolding, pointing out faults, instructions to 'get a grip', comparisons with other people who are better and other criticisms are all types of communication that your voice-hearer is getting anyway from their voices. Try not to become classified as one more critical voice.

Some common but mistaken beliefs that I have come across in carers are:

- It's the cannabis and/or ecstasy and/or cocaine and/or alcohol that caused it.
- Bad friends led them up the garden path.
- The person has become learning disabled.
- Boys normally sleep 20 hours per day, don't they?
- My child has had too easy a life, so then this happens.
- Because they never did drugs before they are not doing it now.
- None of the children in this school do drugs or develop mental health problems.
- My child is defying the family rules.
- All they need is medication.
- Most kids self-harm these days.
- Most young people drink.
- Most young people use common street drugs.
- It's our fault.

First, no single person, group of persons, chemical or event is to blame or caused your child to start hearing voices. Dealing effectively with the situation cannot be about blame. Some or all of these conditions could have contributed in some measure to the complex cocktail that expresses as hearing voices. Add to this an underlay of key developmental stages, single and unexpected traumatic events, personality and genetic vulnerabilities among others and you can see that hearing voices is made up of an intricate tapestry of personal events and circumstances. Consequently, these events are also more or less specific to every voice-hearer.

Routledge
Taylor & Francis Group

No single person, group of persons, chemical or event is to blame.

To address some of the other myths, let me say, first, that your son or daughter has not become learning disabled as a result of hearing voices.

Second, neither boys nor girls sleep 20 hours per day. However, it is not unknown that a voice-hearer may remain in bed longer, possibly as a way of avoiding the day or facing a confusing world in which they feel they are not coping.

Third, young people are often put under pressure to experiment with drugs. Some continue beyond experimentation and will most probably keep that from you, if they have. A claim that it does not happen in a particular school or any other place is inaccurate at the very least. The reality, whether we like it or not, is that drug use among young people does take place. That does not mean that it is acceptable.

Fourth, a person hearing troublesome voices may or may not need medication. However, some form of formal intervention is indicated.

Fifth, most kids do not self-harm, but some do. They do this for a variety of reasons. Self-harming does not necessarily indicate a mental health problem; however, some kind of intervention is needed to help the person break the habit.

Lastly, you are not to blame. This is not about blame.

Remember, too, that Romme (1998) indicated a progression of change. Thus, if the work is put in, this progressive change may look something like this:

1 Initially, your voice-hearer will be fearful and anxious and will show a need to escape. They may also try to escape into a variety of activities. They are still startled by their voices.
2 They may then start investigating what the voices mean to them and start approaching the voices as if they were real people.
3 Finally, they may start accepting themselves, exploring what they were trying to escape from, and not trying to escape any more.

Routledge
Taylor & Francis Group

Progressing through these stages may also show as reengaging with social and occupational activities. It is interesting to note that Romme (1998) nowhere indicates that the voices are gone, even in the final stage. The process has been about learning to deal with voices so that the voice-hearer can get on with their lives, in spite of the voices.

> *There is no magic trick to remove the voices; the trick is for the voice-hearer to get to a point where they do not mind their voices any more.*

4.3 The relationship has changed – what should I do?

It may seem that there is little you can do to help. Just like clinicians, you may well be seen to be on the other side of the fence by your voice-hearer and treated as if you are 'one of them' – one of the people making life (or a desired new lifestyle) difficult for them. The relationship has changed. This is the first awful truth you need to know, so I will stress it.

> *Your relationship with the person you know has changed.*

One of my friends had a breakdown. He became a totally different person: abusive to me, accusing me of things I had not done, suspicious and contemptuous of anything I said. He did, however, 'come back' from the dark place he had entered, much the same as I had known him. He later confirmed that he had heard voices that warned him about me being a member of the CIA.

Accepting the change needs to be part of your point of departure. Accepting the change does not mean agreeing with it, or liking it. It also does not mean giving up. It means clearing the table of stuff that is going to get in the way.

Trying to live in a world that no longer exists will cause much heartache. I am asking much of you – specifically, for you to become pragmatic. This means:

> *You need to see things as they are, not as they were and not as you want them to be.*

If I can perhaps add a necessary piece of hope I would say:

> *This is the way things are now; future change is not impossible.*

Routledge
Taylor & Francis Group

As a clinician, I personally have to believe this, or treatment would be palliative only; thus, I would ask you to work with me on this one. I did this job because I believe in the potential for people to survive and change and overcome bad situations.

I also know that people will not change if I apply excessive pressure. However, I also know that no pressure means little or no change.

As a carer you are in a very tricky position as regards applying any kind of pressure. On the one hand, you know some pressure is necessary but you also know, sometimes through bitter experience, that pressure is quite counterproductive.

If it is your son or daughter we are talking about, you will probably have a natural backlog of communication with them, perhaps without knowing it. So, in effect, the parenting role is probably not a good vehicle to use when approaching your child, simply because for a voice-hearer it may sound too much like a troublesome voice. Some clients have already said to me that they can sometimes not distinguish between what their parents are saying and what the voices are saying. This is understandable and particularly so if the voices are active at the time when you start talking.

Your son or daughter may also now be doing things of which you totally disapprove, for example, taking drugs. It is extremely difficult not to say something that sounds like a criticism or a demand in this type of situation. On the other hand, keeping quiet may seem to you as if you are approving the new behaviour. A key element in working with any person who is using drugs is to engage with them.

> **Engaging with this new person is essential.**

4.4 What should I do about engaging?

When something really bad happens to a person the chances are that they will change in some way. This is true for most of us. It does not mean that this change is bad. What it does mean, however, is that the person has changed and that you need to get to know this changed person.

Thus, one of the most important targets in this new relationship is to try to get to know the person for whom you are the carer, your voice-hearer. This is effectively a relationship you are

Routledge
Taylor & Francis Group

starting anew from this point. Your task is the same as any clinician who wants to work with any client; the first task is to engage.

Engaging means softly, softly forward. It means getting to understand and know this 'new' person without being patronising. You are trying to establish a relationship. You are not trying to re-establish anything, as that would imply you have a plan – a blueprint – of what should emerge at the end of the process.

> *Relating to a changed person means that you should be wary of trying to interact with this person as if they were the old person you knew.*

The aim of engaging is to establish trust in the relationship. During the process of therapy I had to repeat engaging several times with some clients after I had stumbled on to sore toes. I had hurt, scared or angered them unwittingly and this damaged their trust in the relationship. I had become pushy and over-confident; I was now paying the price as my client withdrew from me. The softly, softly, listening posture had to start again. I would expect that you may find you also have to keep engaging.

Engaging is like a dance, matching in counter-point your actions to the other's movements, in this case your voice-hearer.

I found some good pointers for engagement in a booklet produced by the The Sainsbury Centre for Mental Health (2003).

Bear in mind:

- Your voice-hearer may be nervous and wary.
- Their ability to process information may be affected.
- Take them seriously; they are not imagining or faking anything.
- Respect their viewpoint even if it sounds strange to you. Respecting someone's viewpoint does not mean that you necessarily agree with their viewpoint.
- Try to identify common ground.
- Try to be helpful, flexible and active.
- Take stock of how you are presenting to this person. Are you very anxious or analytical or disbelieving? Are you getting frustrated and angry?
- Don't rush getting information. Build the relationship.
- The relationship should be safe for both of you.

The above points represent the rhythms that you have to dance to. If you look at them, they really are not strange; it is pretty much the stuff of any new relationship.

Perhaps the points may sound a bit like you have to submerge yourself entirely. This is certainly not true and should never happen. In fact you, the person, needs to come out in a consistent form. This is extremely important. As Shakespeare wrote in *Hamlet*, 'This above all: to thine own self be true' (1962 [1603], p875). In fact, your voice-hearer needs to have predictable people around them. We all need predictability and this is particularly so in relationships. If I am scared and anxious, predictability in those around me helps me to cope better. If you keep changing like a chameleon it will confuse and agitate your voice-hearer further. It is difficult to marry these two concepts – on the one hand, dancing with your voice-hearer, while, on the other, not losing yourself. Under these conditions:

- You may find it necessary to frequently review your own boundaries and needs.
- You may discover that you need to take a look at your likes, dislikes and principals and then decide which are the ones on which you will not bend, which are stones in your path and which are the ones you have only been mechanically carrying on from family and other norms.
- You may need to figure out what some of your choices and behaviours are costing you.
- You may discover that you need to become aware of your sensitivities and the soft places in your own personality as well as trying to discover your strengths. You may find it useful to discuss this topic with a good friend who is prepared to be honest with you. We all have vulnerabilities and they tend to pop up at those times when we just need to keep a clear head and act purposefully. My vulnerabilities at times cause me to act in ways that are not helpful to the other person, and, in the end, unhelpful to me. This is not about trampling your vulnerabilities; it is about acting on them in a considered way. Be kind to yourself as well.

Once you have a clearer picture of how you are now, you have then discovered your point of departure. Naturally, this knowledge will never come in some moment of divine clarity. We most often learn who we are by bumping into things. Thus, as you learn who you are in this new situation, you will have to update your view of yourself.

In getting to know a changed person, you will need to get to know yourself better.

In the process of getting to know yourself within this new relationship you will find that negotiation skills are an important and necessary part of your new approach. This will affect not

Routledge
Taylor & Francis Group

only living with your voice-hearer, but also with the other people around you. I will give you a short picture of what I have learned about negotiating.

> **In order to negotiate, you have to be prepared to give up something.**

When this particular penny dropped for me, it came as quite a shock. I thought I knew it all and thus was not flexible about giving up anything. I somehow believed that I could out-manoeuvre the person so that they would end up seeing things my way. I quickly learned that if I was going to enter a negotiation with a fixed view of what the outcome has to be, I was wasting my time. Beyond being a waste of time I also learned that being rigid in a negotiation could actually inflict some damage on the relationship.

Therefore, before entering any negotiation see yourself and them as being on opposite hills. Both you and the others are in your castles, weapon and flag in hand, overlooking the valley. In order to negotiate, you all have to leave the safety of your castles as a first step. Everyone has to set aside the protection that old roles, rules and views provided and walk down into the valley – the area of differences between you.

Here are some points that may help you when negotiating:

- To show good will, you may have to leave your castle first.

- Leave the weapons in the castle.

- Leave the flag (attitude) in the castle; better still, leave it in a museum. There may be a new flag when you come back from the negotiation.

- When things get hot (and they probably will), don't run back to the castle; ask for a pause. You need to suck in some fresh air.

- Agree to return.

- Return.

- Try giving choices more than instructions.

- Don't point; someone will bite your finger.

- Speak only for yourself. Use 'I'. Using 'you' is a kind of pointing.

- Give up being an expert.

- Recognise the expertise of the other; the other person will be making some sense. Perhaps it is you who does not understand.

- If you do not understand, ask. Never assume.

- Remember, walking away from a negotiation will end it.

Now that you have some idea of how you should stand, dance and negotiate, let us turn to the voices themselves.

4.5 What should I do with my voice-hearer's voices?

If you like, have a look in the clinician section in 'Practical stuff' in Chapter 3 (section 3.3). What is being said there mostly applies to what you do with your voice-hearer. However, because I do not want to flood you with clinical jargon I will repeat and rephrase some important aspects for your role as a carer.

View the voice as if it is a real flesh and blood person, without ever losing the 'as if'.

After having digested this, remember:

- Your voice-hearer is a new person in your life; they just look like someone you knew.
- They are in a relationship with something that you can neither see nor hear. This relationship is characterised by a struggle for dominance.
- Your voice-hearer has been losing this struggle up to now.
- They need your help to regain an equal position in relationships. Tread carefully; you need their unspoken consent and cooperation to do this.

When you have adopted the view that your voice-hearer is in combat with something, you will notice a few qualities of this battle.

You may discover a common paradox, which at first will confuse you.

Your voice-hearer actually grants power to their voice.

As time goes by you may start getting the impression that a lot of the 'powerful' qualities of the

Routledge
Taylor & Francis Group

voice are reflections of what are the opposite qualities in your voice-hearer. Your voice-hearer's responses cement the relationship as a one-up–one-down set of transactions. You will see that the forcefulness of the voice is met with a deferential or one-down response from your voice-hearer: the shouting and screaming of the voice is met with a terrified silence and the questions posed and demands made by the voice are seldom met with debate or argument. Further, when your voice-hearer eventually tries to regain control it is in an explosion (or implosion) and one possibly of fairly large proportions. A person who screams and shouts as a way of trying to negotiate is out of control, that is, has lost control. By imploding I mean that the person shuts down, disappears into themselves and becomes unreachable and thus more vulnerable.

> **_Exploding or imploding is not a way of getting equal with anyone._**

Although being around a voice-hearer may seem a fraught business, for me Romme's (1998) findings provide hope and help in this area. His discovery suggests that among voice-hearers there are those who have learned to cope with their voices. This is where the magic lies. What we are all trying to do is to get a voice-hearer who is not coping with their voices to shift their position into the coping group.

It is from here that you can take your lead and where you can have an impact. Romme found:

- **Those who cope have proved, and therefore know, that the voices are not so powerful.** By looking at their voices and trying out certain strategies they have noted that their voices are not really that powerful after all. In fact, the belief about the power of voices really only needs a small wedge of doubt to start this process. Just as an example, it is astounding how many voice-hearers are actually scoring a hit on their voices without recognising it. I had to point this out to them often. In a real case I once asked a voice-hearer how many times per week his voice was telling him to kill himself. He corrected me by saying it was more like several times per minute. My first reaction was shock and then it struck me that nowhere on this person's record was there any mention of even attempted self-harm. I pointed this out to him and I could almost see this reality dawning on him. I then added that if the instructions were coming several times per minute and he was not attempting it in some form, this meant that he was successfully resisting the commands several times per minute as well.

- **It is also common that those who are coping had learned to see their voices in a different light.** Perhaps because of the overtly ill will of voices, voice-hearers seldom look

Ⓡ Routledge
Taylor & Francis Group

for neutral or even 'good' voices or even neutral comments by their voice; often because they expect bad, they hear bad. I recall a client who told me of the arrival of a new voice, which I must say dismayed me at the time, but it is not uncommon. I questioned him about the qualities of this voice and was told that it was the voice of a loved but deceased relative and that this person was gently telling him not to be so hard on himself. A good voice, no less. Although I leave good voices alone, I do check up on them from time to time as good voices – like any person – can turn nasty sometimes and be difficult. As regards the bad voices, you could look into understanding who they are. Get a profile of them. Get an idea of the degree of badness. Check up from time to time – as opportunity allows – if that particular voice is still *as* bad. If it is not, ask your voice-hearer how they have changed that by themselves. Do not accept that it is circumstance. Your job, then, is to help them to reduce or erode the degree of 'badness' that they attach to their experience.

- **Those who manage, experience what their voices say typically as statements or opinions and seldom as commands.** I suppose that if we are going to treat voices as real people then we should accept that they, too, are entitled to an opinion. An opinion is not a command and is not always accurate. Your voice-hearer will, for various reasons, unfortunately hear what their voice says as the truth and/or as a command. Perhaps this happens through association. If I say 'I don't like your hat' and I happen to sound like a dominating teacher you had at school, it may sound like I am strongly suggesting that you take the hat off or even get rid of it. It is important that you help your voice-hearer towards a more down-to-earth view of things and limit or transform the associations that they are attaching to the message. I have learned that the colours in which my client paints the voice come from another time and another place. There is nothing strange or 'abnormal' about this process – we all do it; it is merely damaging to self-worth – and we should not all keep on doing it.

- **Further, in dealing with voices those who cope attempt to conduct an assertive conversation with their voices and also to set limits as to the influence the voices have in the relationship.** This is very important. The one-sidedness of the relationship with the voices has to be brought to an end. It is time for your voice-hearer to answer back. Of great importance here is that your voice-hearer remains calm; there should be no shouting, no cursing and no abuse at the voices. Effing and blinding at a voice – as in any relationship – means that the one doing it has lost the battle. Your voice-hearer should not do things that are going to cause them to lose any battle with their voices. Should they lose these battles, you certainly will get your voice-hearer saying to you that talking back 'did not work'. It also

Routledge
Taylor & Francis Group

depends what they were expecting. If they were expecting their voice to immediately and happily engage in a conversation, this would have been unrealistic; no one does that. You need to point out that the aim of the exercise is not for the voice-hearer to become a dictator; you cannot force a person (or a voice) to talk if they do not want to. The aim of the exercise is actually for them to move from being passive in the relationship to establishing a more active, interactional role. In fact, the aim is for them to become the active one, the one who makes the choices about when, what and how they are going to act. People who have a dog or a horse as a pet will quickly understand the reasoning here.

- **Those who cope communicate fairly often about their voices.** Voice-hearers do not easily talk about their voices for many reasons. Imagine a voice to be like a crime boss who is threatening you with hellfire, death and damnation. You, too, would not easily talk freely about this voice. The voice is an experience that holds nothing good for your voice-hearer. It is extremely scary and the threats sound real and close at hand. Some voices will even issue threats about the person with whom they have discussed their voice. Thus, your voice-hearer's voice may even turn their attention to your safety! I have had that happen; the client I was with suddenly said, 'Joe (the voice) has just said he can read your mind and will put thoughts into your head.' I must admit that – for a second – I felt a chill. It felt as if 'Big Brother' was listening. Further, many voice-hearers strongly believe that the voice can actually physically harm them or, alternatively, force them to harm themselves. Harming themselves is a risk when the voice instructs them to do so and this should be born in mind. However, you cannot watch your voice-hearer all the time. One avenue I have used in cases like this is to analyze what the voice is 'commanding' my client to do and try to find suitable ways of them punching holes in the command itself. However, this is not foolproof. There is no foolproof way of dealing with the threat of self-harm. Beyond this specific issue, you can also point out to your voice-hearer that when they talk about their voices there is not always a negative effect. Remember, your voice-hearer counts the failures and the bad events rather than the successes and the neutral or good events. You may have to help them to get a more balanced picture.

- **Those who achieve equality with their voices commonly use focusing (non-avoidance) strategies.** Distraction (avoidance) has little if any value. Listening to music turned up loud or abusing substances certainly has no long-term value at all. At best, these strategies are like a tourniquet; when it comes off, the problem returns. The voice-hearer needs to be helped to abandon avoidance as a strategy.

Routledge
Taylor & Francis Group

By now, you will have got the idea about what a 'focusing' strategy is. It is grasping the nettle and holding on for as long as that can be tolerated; it is doing battle and retreating, but never abandoning the struggle. It is spending the appropriate amount of time talking about it in order to actively analyze it and seek ways of engaging with it in the most effective way. It also means actively acknowledging success in a non-boastful or patronising way.

> *The relationship your voice-hearer has with voices is all about being dominated and being unequal.*

Remember, too, that in helping your voice-hearer you also should not dominate or harass; you must avoid becoming like the voices. Tread softly with small steps. Be patient. Be gentle.

If your voice-hearer found these practices difficult in their ordinary lives before hearing voices, it explains a lot. They will need to change merely in order to get through life without too many scars anyway.

> *Many of the changes voice-hearers make towards their voices are also necessary changes in their general relationships.*

> *Expect to be shocked when your voice-hearer starts coping with their voices; they will probably change toward you as well.*

I remember this happening to me in a therapy session. I had been treating a very unassertive person (not a voice-hearer). Therapy had gone on for several sessions of assertiveness training. It felt like I was getting nowhere. Then, one day I was a few minutes late in starting the session and my client tackled me about it. This was a very different person that was talking to me now! When I pointed that out to her, she chastised me with a twinkle in her eye, asking if I expected her to go on being unassertive with me. I should have seen that coming if I believed in my own therapy. This person had not changed overnight from unassertive to assertive; unseen changes had been slowly embedding themselves and then, at a particular opportunity, the person took their new skills into full practice.

> *When changes occur in a person, they often do so unseen and over a period of time. Changes may appear apparently 'out of the blue'.*

Routledge
Taylor & Francis Group

> *Changes in any person can occur when new meanings and interpretations are attached to old experiences and relationships.*

In Chapter 3 I spoke quite freely about interpretation or the meaning that all of us attach to experiences, but have not dealt with it here – from a carer's perspective – yet.

To start off we need the quote by Nietzsche at the front of the book: 'There are no facts, only interpretations.' This is an extremely important concept to bear in mind when dealing with voice-hearing. I must, however, stress that Nietzsche did not mean that we fabricate facts; it means that each of us has a unique filter, if you wish, through which all our senses are squeezed. The end product is what each of us sees, hears, smells, tastes and senses.

Let me illustrate this with an example. Let us say that I know very little about snakes. Should someone then throw a snake into the room, I may well jump on to the nearest table. Why? It is because I am assuming that all snakes are dangerous, for a start. In other words, I have interpreted the experience as dangerous. Now, if I was an expert on snakes, I may even walk up to it knowing that this particular snake, being a brown egg eater, is not a problem.

My knowledge of snakes will drastically influence the meaning I place on it. An interpretation that suggests risk will have an entirely different set of consequences to an interpretation that registers no or low risk.

> *As your voice-hearer gets to know more about their voices, they will fear them less.*

Thus, if there is any way you can assist your voice-hearer to get to know their voices better, it will be of much use to them. However, never force them to talk about their voices; they will soon shut that topic down if there is stress associated with it.

Further, helping your voice-hearer to gain greater insight into their voices could parallel what a good general does. A good general will always gather information about the enemy: its weak points, common positioning and tactics and weaknesses in its organisation (such as clashes within its activities). These types of weakness are then exploited almost as a wedge to split the enemy apart. If your voice-hearer is talking to you about his or her voices then you have the

103

opportunity to gather intelligence on the voices and how they operate. By being party to this knowledge will very likely provide you with useful information that can be used against the voices.

Clinical example

My group co-facilitator and I discovered an extremely interesting case of how a voice achieved control over a client. This happened mainly because the person had not put two and two together on what the voice was doing but rather responded impulsively with anger. Bear in mind what controlling means; if I am controlling you it means that I get you to do something that I want you to do.

This particular client had an in-depth knowledge of the bible. From time to time his voice would make an inaccurate statement about something that was in the bible. The person could not leave it at that; he used to spend hours arguing with his voice. On the surface he was doing what we had asked him to do: he was being active and assertive in the relationship. However, seen from another perspective, by 'making a mistake' the voice had enticed the person into an argument. Although this may sound a bit fanciful, it is nonetheless another 'hidden' aspect of unassertiveness. If I through my actions suggest that you behave in a certain way and you do it, then I am controlling you. If I look up into the sky with a curious look on my face, it would be hard for you to stop yourself from looking up as well. The client in this case was falling prey to a variation on a well-known interactional game described by Eric Bernes (2010) that I call 'Let's you and me fight'. It is no less than throwing down the gauntlet, which any stout-hearted person would pick up. The point is, however, that often the person doing so is reacting, rather than making a choice. Our ploy was to point this out to the client, urging him to make a choice about what his voice may be suggesting he do. There is nothing wrong in debating, but being tricked into a debate is another matter.

Being controlled often happens at subtle levels.

Thus, with all you have to do, being a family member or a friend of someone who hears voices can be very challenging. Apart from seeing your loved one or friend suffering, your attentions and offers of help will be rejected. You should expect this to happen often, particularly in the beginning. As your voice-hearer reframes the picture they have of you from something that is as

Routledge
Taylor & Francis Group

troublesome as their voice to being a helper, a traveller who is making the journey toward a new life with them, they will become more cooperative. It takes enormous patience and there will be times when you will feel rejected, helpless and useless. As a counter to this, all I can say is that we had a large poster in our team room depicting some water bird swallowing a frog and at the same time the frog was strangling the bird. Its caption read, 'Never give up!'

Routledge
Taylor & Francis Group

Routledge
Taylor & Francis Group

Chapter 5

In conclusion

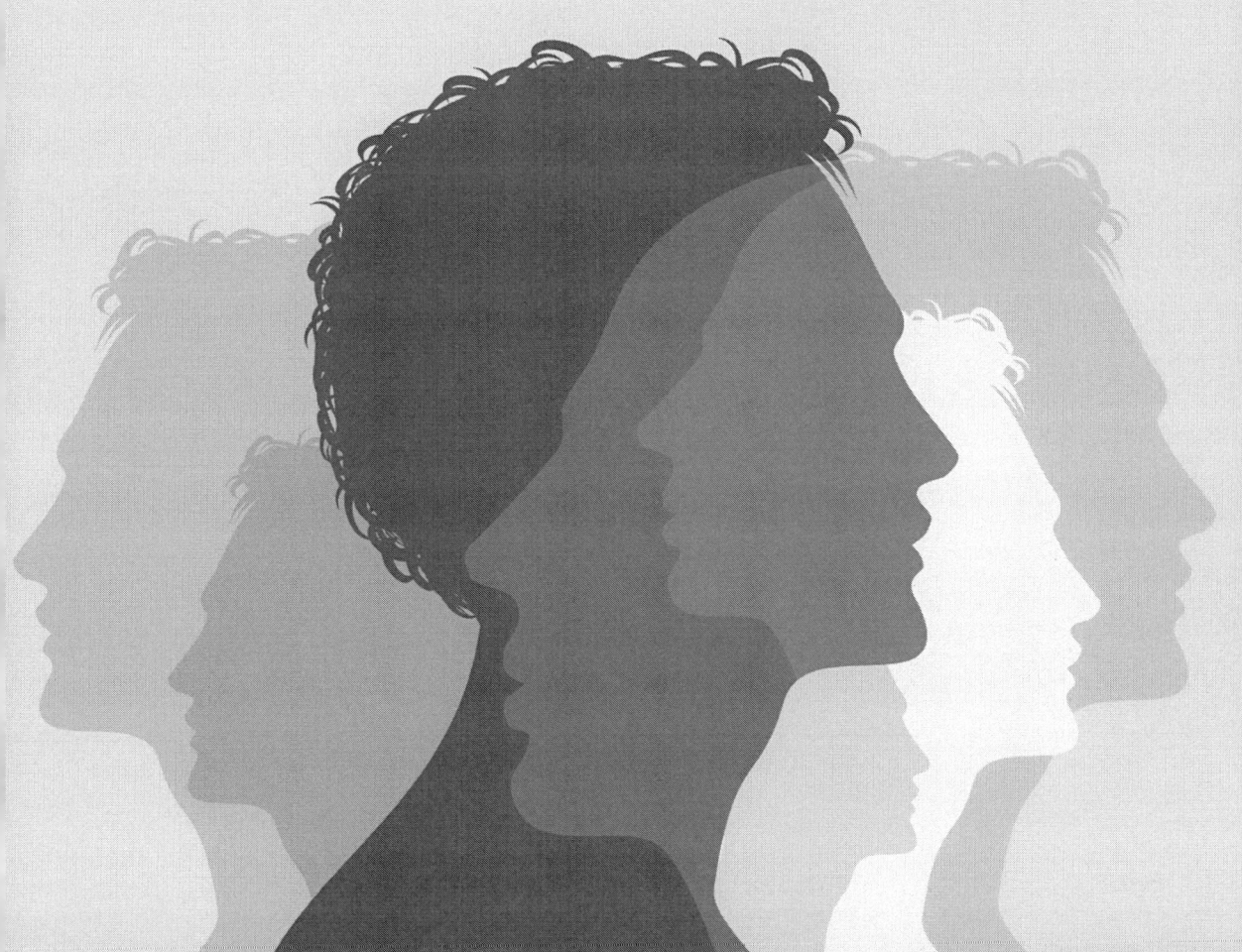

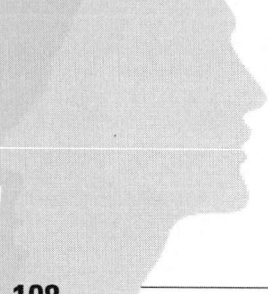

Routledge
Taylor & Francis Group

In conclusion

For those who hear voices it would often seem that the easiest option is to give in and do what the voice says. This pathway may lead to a life of torment, some of it being spent in mental institutions. The options covered in this book do not offer instant salvation; rather they offer the possibility of reward after a period of 'blood, sweat and tears'. It is hard work reversing a process that forced a voice-hearer into submission, but it is worthwhile work.

It is work that will take you into frightening areas in which you seem to be challenging some kind of devil. It is work that is filled with anxiety and apprehension. But, it is work that needs to be done. I once read a book called *I Never Promised You a Rose Garden* (1964). The book was about a voice-hearer. Overcoming voices certainly is not a rose garden. It is, however, so important to hang on in there and never give up. Nothing worthwhile has ever been achieved in a short while or without effort. If things come too easily, they often turn out to be the wrong things.

Then there are those who are trying to help people who experience troublesome voices. You will find it extremely demanding. It requires dedication under severe pressure from the voice-hearers for you to leave them alone. You may be vilified, ignored and even abused by your voice-hearer as they resist your attempts to help. You have to become the extreme strategist, balancing a softly, softly approach while helping your voice-hearer to adopt new (and to them) strange views and behaviours. You also have to cope with what is no less than a new relationship. To cap it all, you have to adopt a 'never give up' attitude.

In spite of the difficulties and the hard work, many have walked this path and have arrived at a point where voices play little if any role in their lives. They have experienced a release from the constraints that their relationship with their voices imposed on them.

Central to these approaches are some guidelines that were among and can be read into what I presented as highlighted key-point text within the different sections. I will outline these guidelines here within the sections in which they were presented.

I truly hope that this book has given you hope and a belief that overcoming voices is possible.

5.1 Guidance notes taken from chapters

From Chapter 1: Approaching the problem of voices

The meanings that voice-hearers attach to their voices play a big role in the way they experience them and thus in the way that they deal with them.

A person who hears voices often believes that their voices are all powerful.

Dealing with voices is similar to dealing with any troublesome relationship.

It is a relationship in which the voice-hearer is being controlled by their voice(s):

- The voice tells the voice-hearer who they are, who they have been and who they will be in the next minute, hour, day or months.
- The voice tells the voice-hearer what to do, how to do it and when to do it. Sometimes this even goes down to how they should walk, what they should say and how they should say it.
- The voice comes and goes as it pleases and when it does this it is telling voice-hearers to pay attention to them, now.

This is a picture of someone who is being dominated all the time. Even when voices are not there, the voice-hearer will be waiting for them, just like in any horror movie.

From Chapter 2: For voice-hearers

Be careful not to give your voice any power. When you think that it has qualities that it does not actually have, you are giving it power.

Changing the way you think about voices. It is thus very important that you think about the following:

- **You are in a relationship with your voices.** Because your voice often conveys a message to you that is more or less understandable and you are able to act on that message in some way, this makes what is happening sound very much like a relationship. The next point takes this definition a step further.
- **These are your voices; nobody else has them**. Other voice-hearers have voices that may be similar but when you get to the detail, they are exclusive to a particular voice-hearer. Just

like a circle of work colleagues or even friends that are exclusively yours, your voices are exclusively yours.

- **Treat the voices as if they are 'real' people**, however crazy this sounds. Remember that this is only 'as if'. You do this to help you understand that you actually have a relationship with them. Only then can you deal with the problems they present to you, as you would with a flesh and blood person.
- **Some people cope with their voices**; it is possible for you to learn to cope with yours as well.
- **Voices are not superpowerful.** If voices were that powerful then nobody would be able to cope with them and nobody would learn *how* to cope with them.

Generally, therefore:

- You should not allow yourself to be dominated or controlled by anyone.
- Avoiding a problem does not solve it.

Your voice cannot be allowed to:

- call the shots
- tell you what to do and how to do it
- turn up at any time and expect you to drop everything to listen to what it has to say
- threaten you
- curse at, swear at and abuse you without a response.

However, your voice can be allowed to:

- have an opinion
- make suggestions
- give you health warnings
- talk to you in a calm way
- approach you rather than gatecrash.

Voices are bullies; you should be firm but not aggressive when dealing with a bully.

If you keep denying that you hear a voice, you will know nothing about it; it will remain a stranger and every time it pitches up you will be startled.

  Routledge
Taylor & Francis Group

When you get to know about something, you fear it less.

Getting to know your voice is like creating a map so that you can see what you are dealing with. Keeping quiet could mean that you agree with what the voice is saying.

The more you stand up and face your voice, the better you will feel within yourself – even if your knees are shaking.

Your voice does not have to answer you. If your voice does not answer, maybe it does not have an answer.

Voices find and highlight your weaknesses, fears and faults.

Why are your voice's remarks so important to you?

Don't play the game that your voice suggests.

Every time you find just one instance when you are not as bad as the voice is saying, you are also finding an instance when your voices are wrong.

Start treating yourself with respect; perhaps the voices will also do that.

Listening and waiting for a scary thing will make you anxious.

There are other things that are more important than your voices.

The 'in spite of' strategy says: I am not going to let what is happening now ruin my day.

You do not have to do what your voice tells you to do, even if you tell your voice that you will do it. What you do is your choice.

If your voice does not do what you request, you have not failed.

Whatever we experience has some personal meaning for us.

Routledge
Taylor & Francis Group

Having a clearer picture of the personal things that drive your life could help you to have more control in many areas.

Voices love it when you crank up your emotions.

Although you may feel like throwing in the towel, never give up.

From Chapter 3: For clinicians

It would seem that:

- A clinician who feels inadequate when working with a certain condition is in an extremely difficult if not depressing situation.
- A clinician who has no techniques to hand will grasp at anything.

Generally, therefore:

We should stop doing things that do not work or that make things worse.

We should start doing things that move towards an outcome of the person coping with their voices.

Avoidance is a short-term strategy that keeps anxiety high and offers no lasting effect.

Avoidance strategies contain powerful conditioning elements through which your voice-hearer may become addicted to avoidance.

Your central area of work lies within the voice-hearer's interpretation of experiences and how they translate this into behaviour.

Ultimately, behaviour should work for rather than against the person.

Working with voice-hearers requires that you examine where you stand on a variety of issues.

When you work with voice-hearers you should be aware that their experiences – past and present – place them at considerable risk.

Voice-hearers are seldom attention seeking. It is best to act on risky warning signs.

Routledge
Taylor & Francis Group

It is helpful when as many of those who work with voice-hearers understand the experiences that voices-hearers have.

You will need to be prepared to view a voice-hearer and the idea of voice-hearing in a way that is free from dogma.

Whenever an avoidance strategy is stopped the immediate effect is often that the voices become worse in some way.

Avoiding a problem does not solve it.

Offering a strategy that suggests your client should put their head in the sand will cause them to get their butts kicked.

It would be useful to get a working knowledge of a variety of approaches.

From Chapter 4: For carers and family

In many cases troublesome voices can be overcome to varying degrees.

Being made aware that someone close to you is hearing voices may cause a reaction that looks a lot like grief.

The person you knew may be very different from the one who is now hearing troublesome voices.

No single person, group of persons, chemical or event is to blame.

There is no magic trick to remove the voices; the trick is for the voice-hearer to get to a point where they do not mind their voices any more.

Your relationship with the person you know has changed.

You need to see things as they are, not as they were and not as you want them to be.

Routledge
Taylor & Francis Group

This is the way things are *now*, future change is not impossible.
Engaging with this new person is essential.

Relating to a changed person means that you should be wary of trying to interact with this person as if they were the old person you knew.

In getting to know a changed person, you will need to get to know yourself better.

Negotiating may become an important process in this new relationship. In order to negotiate, you have to be prepared to give up something.

View the voice as if it is a real flesh and blood person, without ever losing the 'as if'.

Your voice-hearer:

- is clearly in a relationship with something that you can neither see nor hear and this relationship is characterised by a struggle for dominance
- has been losing this struggle up to now
- needs your help to regain an equal position in relationships; tread carefully in this as you need their unspoken consent and cooperation to do this.

Your voice-hearer actually grants power to their voice.

The relationship your voice-hearer has with voices is all about being dominated and being unequal.

Exploding or imploding is not a way of getting equal with anyone.

Many of the changes voice-hearers make towards their voices are also necessary changes in their general relationships.

Expect to be shocked when your voice-hearer starts coping with their voices; they will probably change toward you as well.

When changes occur in a person, they often do so unseen and over a period of time. Changes may appear apparently 'out of the blue'.

Changes in any person can occur when new meanings and interpretations are attached to old experiences and relationships.

As your voice-hearer gets to know more about their voices, they will fear them less.

Being controlled often happens at subtle levels.

Don't ever give up!

Routledge
Taylor & Francis Group

Appendices

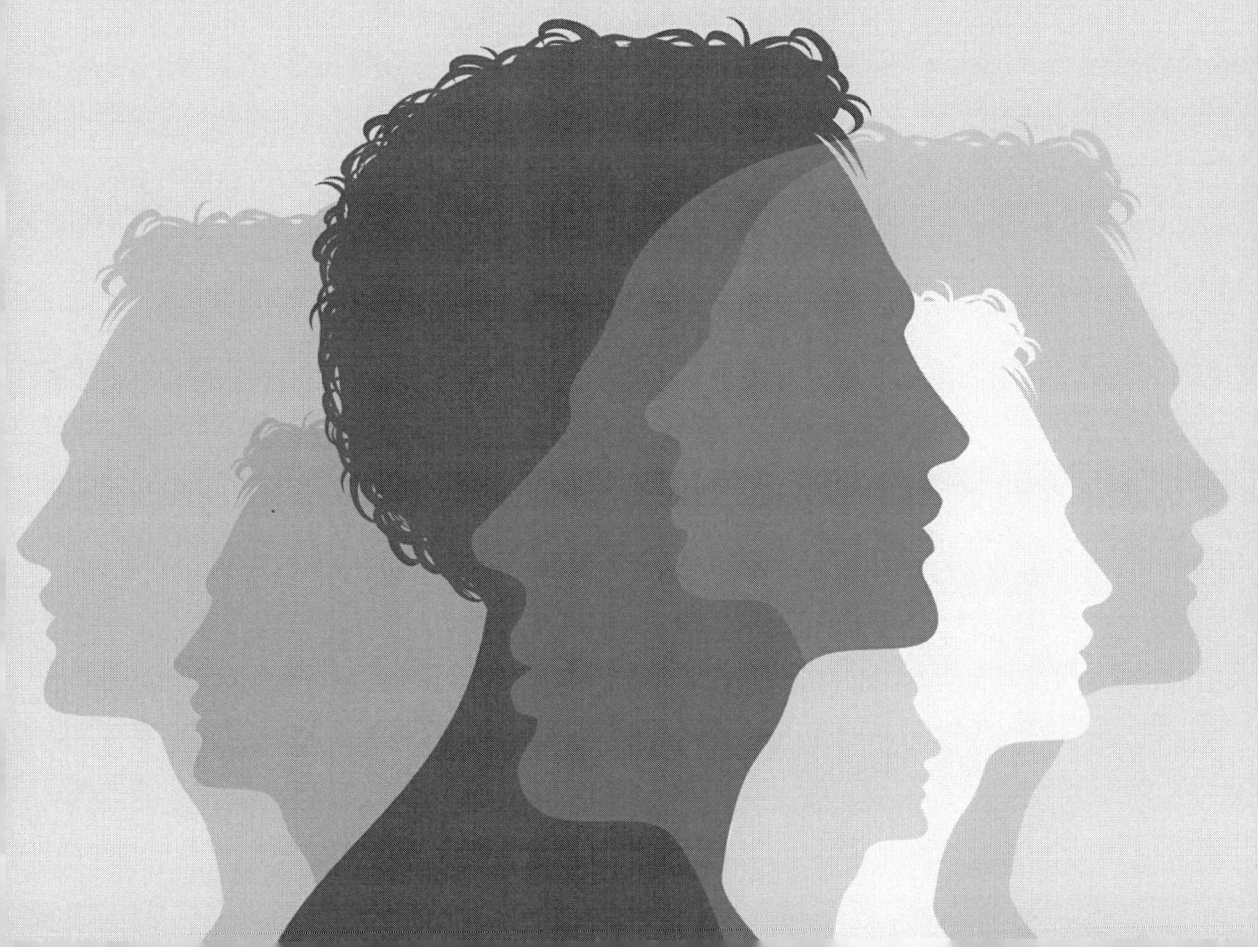

Routledge
Taylor & Francis Group

Appendix 1: Self-worth

- Self-worth is what I think about myself.
- Self-worth is not what others think of me; that's why it's called *self*-worth.

My self-worth depends on:

- recognising when I get something right
- saying 'thanks' to myself from time to time
- saying 'hello' to myself from time to time
- recognising my achievements, however small
- asking myself what I want from time to time
- praising myself when it's due
- looking for the good in me
- daring to be myself
- putting myself equal to (not above or below) others
- not always criticising myself
- taking actions to try to fix it when I find fault with something that I have done
- accepting that others may be different to me but that they are not really better than I am
- treating myself with respect.

R Routledge
Taylor & Francis Group

Appendix 2: Assertiveness

- Assertiveness is a skill; no one is born assertive. Like any skill, it can be learned. Like any skill, it needs to be practised in order for it to become part of a person's 'survival kit'. If it is not practised, it will become rusty.

- Assertive statements often begin with the word 'I'. Avoid using finger pointing as seen in 'you' type statements. 'You' statements are open to challenge and debate. Definitive statements about yourself are not really open to debate.

- Assertive statements are not aggressive. Aggression is a sign of unassertiveness.

- Assertive statements cover the full range of communication; from as little as clearly and unambiguously asking for a railway ticket at the railway station to correcting another person about the way they see you and/or want you to be.

- Being assertive may involve repeating your stance. Naturally, the person may not agree with you; they also have a right to an opinion and to be assertive.

The definition of assertiveness as developed at The Byron Day Care Unit (Tindal Centre, Aylesbury, Buckinghamshire, in the 1990s): 'Assertiveness involves standing up for your rights without ignoring the rights of others ... Assertiveness incorporates the idea of respect for oneself and for others – respect which allows requests and demands to be refused if inappropriate, which does not apply pressure and which leaves room for compromise.'

Routledge
Taylor & Francis Group

Appendix 3: Strategic overview

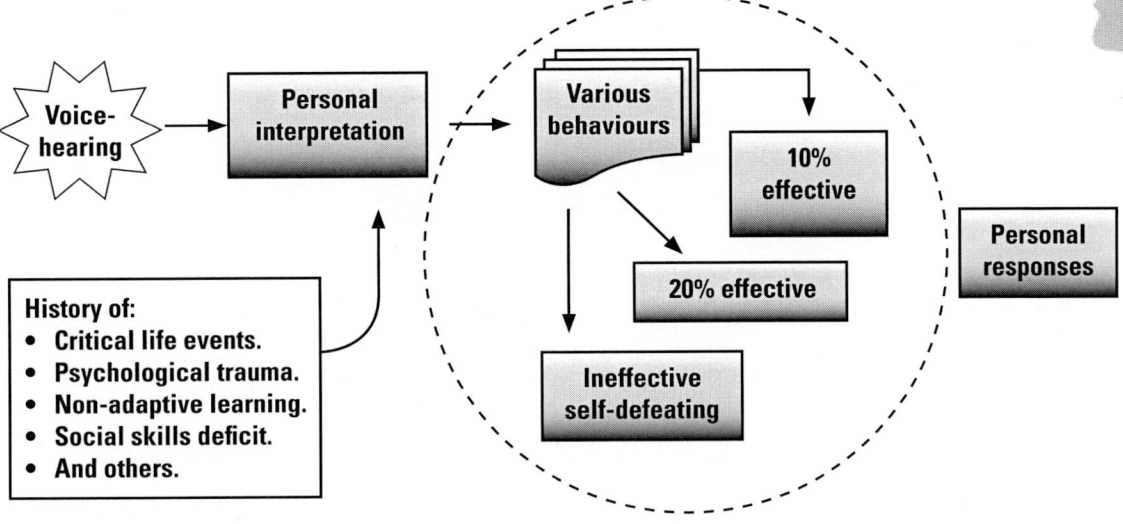

Targets for therapy
Content targets (information, the 'WHAT'):

- Life narrative/history.
- Personal interpretation.
- Personal responses – what are they?
- What is the effect of the response; does it work in any way at all, or does it primarily have a negative outcome?

Process targets (therapeutic tasks, the 'HOW', detecting and analysing PATTERNS of response and changing the non-productive patterns into productive patterns)

Empowerment through:

- Breaking the person's isolation with their voice hearing experience.
- Encouraging the person to form an assertive dialogue with their voices.
- Discovering the person's unique response repertoire to their experience of hearing voices. How is the person achieving the outcome that is evident?
- Identify unproductive and self-defeating strategies used by the person.
- Identify, highlighting and building upon those strategies which are productive (However small).
- Reframing automatic negative thoughts which underpin potentially unproductive/self-defeating responses towards the voice-hearing experience.
- Challenging misperceptions, misinterpretations, myths and dysfunctional beliefs that underpin the qualities the person assigns to the voice-hearing experience.
- Client centred, collaborative.
- Encouraging the development of the person's own (internal) frame of reference.

Appendix 4: Emergencies flowchart

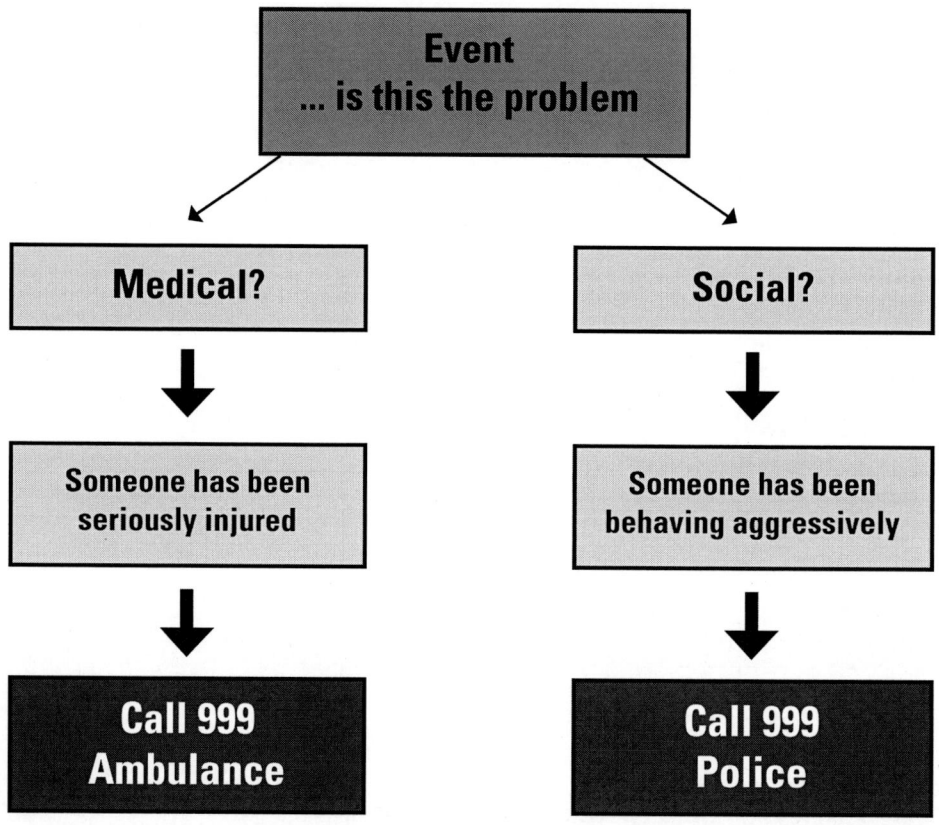

```
                    ┌─────────────────────────────┐
                    │           Event             │
                    │   ... is this the problem   │
                    └─────────────────────────────┘
                        ↙                     ↘
        ┌──────────────────┐          ┌──────────────────┐
        │     Medical?     │          │     Social?      │
        └──────────────────┘          └──────────────────┘
                 ↓                              ↓
        ┌──────────────────┐          ┌──────────────────┐
        │ Someone has been │          │ Someone has been │
        │ seriously injured│          │behaving aggressively│
        └──────────────────┘          └──────────────────┘
                 ↓                              ↓
        ┌──────────────────┐          ┌──────────────────┐
        │     Call 999     │          │     Call 999     │
        │     Ambulance    │          │      Police      │
        └──────────────────┘          └──────────────────┘
```

IF SOMEONE HAS BEEN SERIOUSLY INJURED,
CALL AMBULANCE FIRST, THEN POLICE IF NECESSARY

Routledge
Taylor & Francis Group

Appendix 5: Patsy Hage's story

Patsy Hage, one of Marius Romme's patients (and co-founder of the hearing voices movement), had a substantial history of hearing very destructive voices. It was while working with her that Romme came on the idea of a new approach to treating voice-hearers.

Because she was so desperate, Patsy did a lot of research into voice-hearing.

Up to this point, she had been treated with a range of medications that had no effect on reducing any quality of the voices themselves. Although the medications did reduce anxiety, they also interfered with her concentration. During this time she became depressed and suicidal. Romme was at his wit's end and, in desperation, gave her a book by Julian Jayne entitled *The Origins of Consciousness and the Breakdown of the Bicameral Mind*.

Patsy had never believed that she suffered from any illness and from Jayne's book she deduced that in certain cases hearing voices was considered normal. She confronted Romme about this, because, on reflection, she found that she was angry with him because he had never asked her about what the voices were saying to her. Apparently, she said to him: 'You believe in a God we never see or hear, so why shouldn't you believe in the voices I really do hear?'

At this time, Romme had held the standard view of voices as being part of a mental illness. Her reasoning made sense to him and he changed his working style with her.

Once they had started exploring her whole experience of voice-hearing, a lot of things started falling into place for Romme . For example, her voices, which at first were friendly, started soon after a traumatic event when she was eight years old. However, in her mid-teens the voices became negative.

Patsy's persistence in finding an alternative way of managing voices, as well as her proving to Marius Romme that other ways are possible and effective, ushered in a new perspective to dealing with voices.

Source: adapted from Intervoice.

Ɍ Routledge
Taylor & Francis Group

Appendix 6: My history of hearing voices

1 When did you first hear voices? How old were you?

....

2 What was happening at the time you heard your first voice?

....
....
....
....

3 If you hear more than one voice, which one came first?

....

4 If you hear more than one voice, when did the others arrive?

....
....
....
....

5 Have your voices changed in any way?

....
....
....
....

6 What do you think made them change?

....
....
....
....

Routledge
Taylor & Francis Group

7   Is there anything that triggers your voices?

....

....

....

....

8   What sorts of things make your voices worse?

....

....

....

....

R Routledge
Taylor & Francis Group

Appendix 7: Voices rap sheet

If you get tired or too anxious doing this, stop. Continue later.

1   How many voices do you hear? ....

2   Do any of them have names? If so, what are their names?

3   Which of these is the strongest and which is the weakest?

.... (strongest) and .... (weakest)

4   What makes one stronger and the other weaker?

....

....

....

5   Do you have any good, helpful and/or friendly voices?

....

....

....

6   Do any of your voices remind you of someone you knew, or know? If so, who?

....

....

Routledge
Taylor & Francis Group

7 Have you heard anywhere before the things that the voices say? If so, where?

....

....

....

8 Do any of your voices sometimes make mistakes?

....

....

....

9 If you were to guess, how do you think your voices are feeling, for example, happy, sad, angry, frustrated or lonely?

....

....

....

10 If you have angry voices, why do you think they are angry?

....

....

....

 Routledge
Taylor & Francis Group

Appendix 8: Strategies that you use to deal with your voices

Date	Strategy What did you do with your voice?	Effect on voices How did the voices respond?	Outcome **How well did this work?** Score out of 10.

Strategies are the things you do to make your voices less threatening or to come less often or speak more softly or be less abusive. In other words, strategies are anything that makes them more bearable.

R Routledge
Taylor & Francis Group

Appendix 9: Getting my life back

What am I doing now that I was struggling with two months ago?

Scoring: 10 = extremely difficult or impossible   0 = extremely easy

Case example:

Activity	Two months ago	Now
I take my dog out two times a day now, whereas taking her out at all was impossible for me two months ago.	10	5
I talk to my voices.	8	5
I took my family out into town when I was very nervous.	10	8
I go shopping.	10	5
I go to a community group every week.	9	7

Activity	Two months ago	Now

Routledge Taylor & Francis Group

Appendix 10: Relapse prevention

Relapse prevention focuses on establishing a general as well as an individualised profile of a relapse pattern or signature where possible. It will also include a 'Relapse Drill' – that is, the specific actions the client could take to try to minimise and halt the progress of relapse.

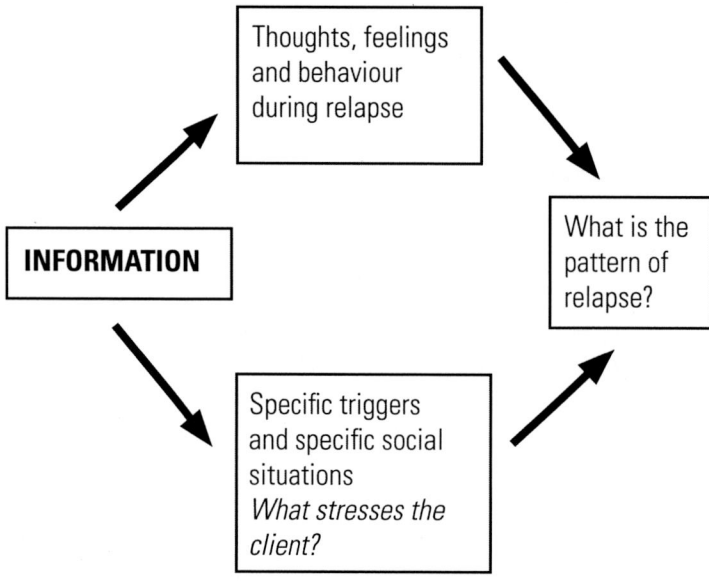

R Routledge
Taylor & Francis Group

References

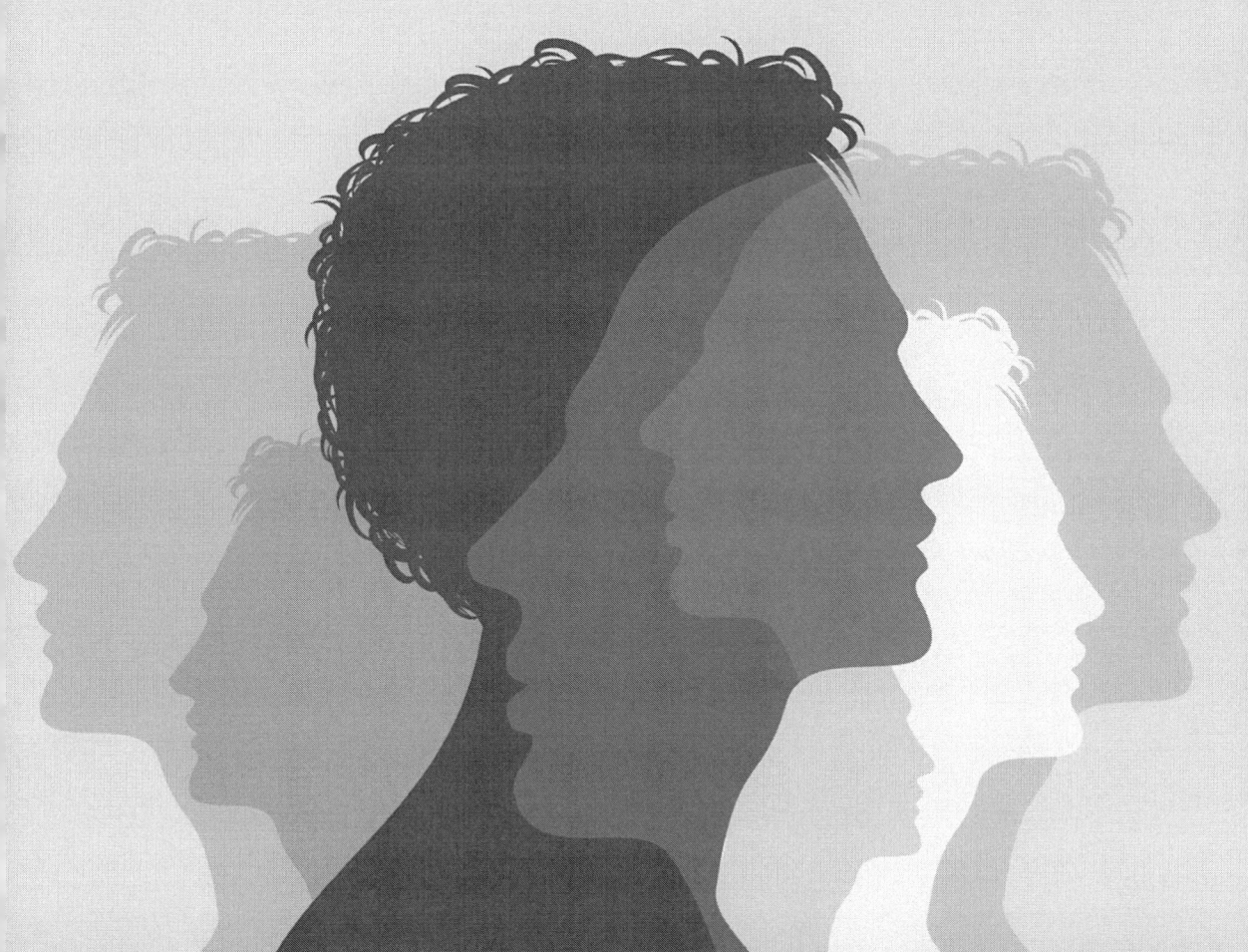

Bernes E (2010) *Games People Play: The Psychology of Human Relationships*, Penguin Books, London.

Birchwood M (2006) Presentation *The Cognitive Model of Distress and Behaviour*, International Early Psychosis Association (IEPA), 5 October, Birmingham.

Buckinghamshire Early Intervention Service (2007a) *Operational Policy*, November.

Buckinghamshire Early Intervention Service (2007b) *Am I OK?*, online, Oxford Health NHS Foundation Trust, www.am-i-ok.co.uk/index.htm (accessed 19 May 2015).

Dorland's Medical Dictionary (2015) *Assertiveness*, Wikipedia entry, online, http://en.wikipedia.org/wiki/Assertiveness (accessed 26 May 2015).

Fadden G, James C & Pinfold V (2012) *Caring for Yourself – Self-help for Families and Friends Supporting People with Mental Health Problems*, White Halo Design, Birmingham.

Festinger L (1957) *A Theory of Cognitive Dissonance*, Stanford University Press, Stanford, CA.

Frusciante J (2010) *Famous People who Hear Voices*, online, www.intervoiceonline.org (accessed October 2010).

Greenberg J (1964) *I Never Promised You a Rose Garden*, St Martin's Paperback, USA.

Haley J (1963) *Strategies of Psychotherapy*, Wiley, New York, NY.

Ingram GCI (2009) *Displacement Activity*, online, http://en.wikipedia.org/wiki/Displacement_activity (accessed April 2015).

Intervoice (2012) *Patsy Hague: Co-founder*, online, www.intervoiceonline.org/about-intervoice/patsy-hague-co-founder (accessed October 2012).

Jeffers S (1991) *Feel the Fear and Do It Anyway*, Arrow Books, London.

  Routledge
Taylor & Francis Group

Maier HW (ed) (1969) *Three Theories of Child Development: Contributions of Erik H. Erikson, Jean Piaget and Robert Sears, and Their Applications,* revised edn, Harper & Row Publishers, New York, NY, Evanston, IL and London.

Maslow AH & Mittelmann B (1951) *Principles of Abnormal Psychology: The Dynamics of Psychic Illness,* Harper Brothers, New York, NY.

McMillen K (1966) *When I Loved Myself Enough,* Sidgwick & Jackson, London.

Nietzsche F (1886–7) *Friedrich Nietzsche,* online, http://en.wikiquote.org/wiki/Friedrich_Nietzsche (accessed 2015).

Oxford Paperback Dictionary, The (1982) Oxford University Press, Oxford.

Powell TJ (1992) 'What starts and maintains anxiety?', *The Mental Health Handbook: A Cognitive Behavioural Approach,* Speechmark Publishing, Brackley.

Romme M (1998) *Understanding Voices – Coping with Auditory Hallucinations and Confusing Realities,* Handsell Publications, Maastricht.

Romme M & Escher S (2000) *Making Sense of Voices,* Mind Publications, London.

Sainsbury Centre for Mental Health, The (2003) *A Window of Opportunity: A Practical Guide for Developing Early Intervention in Psychosis Services,* Sainsbury Centre for Mental Health Publications, London.

Sarason IG (1972) *Abnormal Psychology,* Pearson Education, Upper Saddle River, NJ.

Shakespeare W (1962 [1603]) *The Complete Works of William Shakespeare,* Craig WJ (ed), Oxford University Press, Oxford.

Solly A (2005) 'Mindfulness and cognitive therapy', *Clinical Psychology,* (45), pp10–11.

Sun Tzu (*c.* 500 **BC**) *The Art of War,* online, http://en.wikiquote.org/wiki/Sun_Tzu (accessed 2015).

Routledge
Taylor & Francis Group

von Bertalanffy L (1968) *General System Theory: Foundations, Development, Applications*, revised edn, George Braziller, New York, NY.

Watzlawick P, Beavin JH & Jackson DD (1967) *The Pragmatics of Human Communication*, Norton and co., Toronto.

Watzlawick P, Weakland, JH & Fisch, R (1974) *Change: Principles of Problem Formation and Problem Resolution*, Norton, Oxford.

Yalom ID (1975) *The Theory and Practice of Group Psychotherapy*, 1st edn, Basic Books, New York, NY.

Routledge
Taylor & Francis Group

Routledge
Taylor & Francis Group

Index

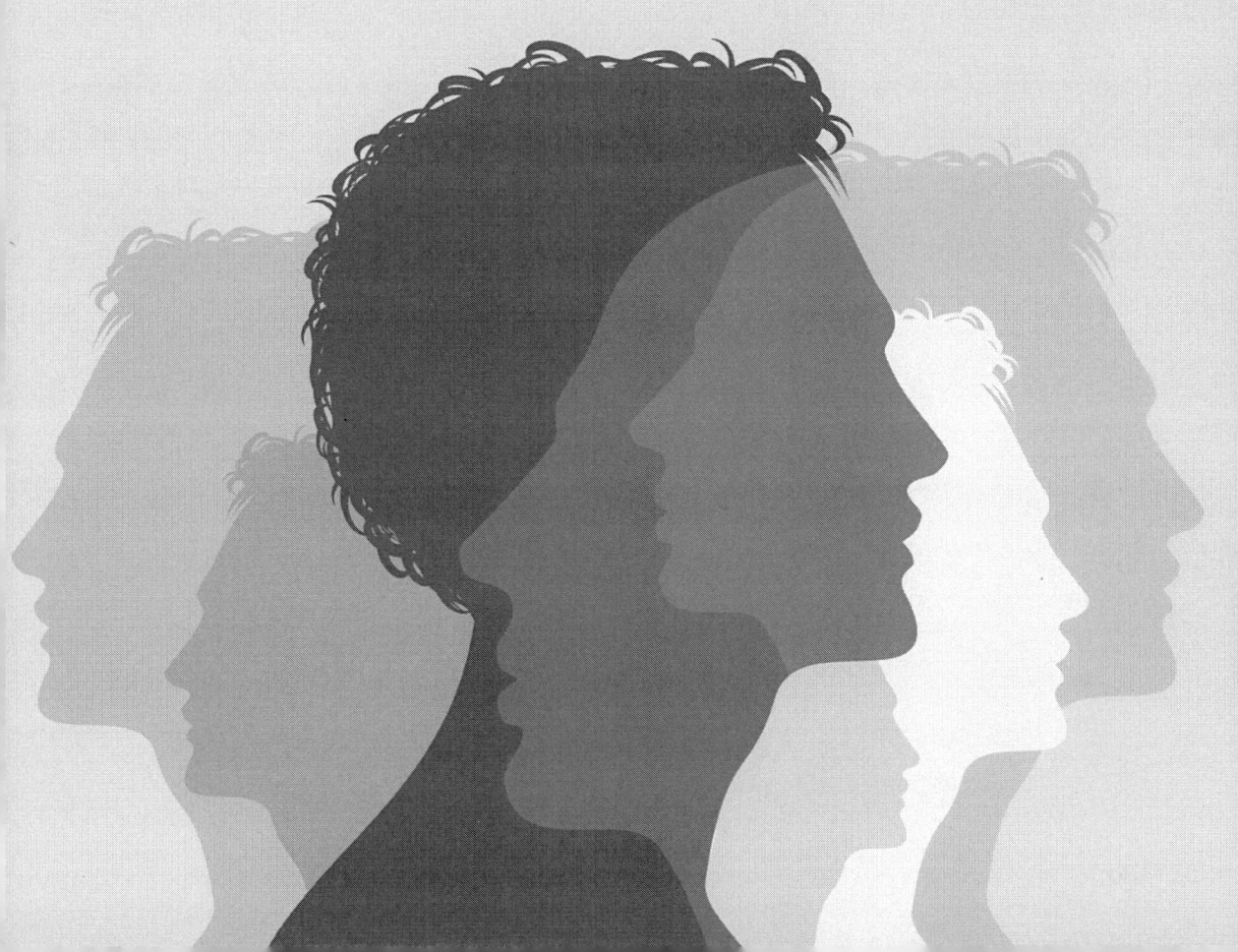

Index

abuse 35, 62, 75

actions 12-20

feelings—thoughts—actions cycle 14-15, 19, 43

alcohol 29, 89

anger 72-3

anomalous experiences 19, 20, 65

anxiety 8, 16-20, 25-7, 59, 70

assertiveness 32-3, 36, 51, 72, 100-1, 102, 120

attitude, clinician's 57-61

automatic negative thoughts 28, 29

autonomic physical responses 27, 59

avoidance strategies 11, 17-19, 55-6, 101

effect of stopping 62-3

focusing vs 70-3

bad voices 54, 99-100

behavioural approaches 65-73

behavioural family therapy 70-1

beliefs 68

carers' mistaken beliefs 91

challenging beliefs about voices 69-70

Bentall, R. 57

bereavement 87

Bernes, E. 104

Birchwood, M. 57, 74

blame 91-2

breakdown 19, 93

Buckinghamshire Early Intervention Service vii, 86

bullying 30-1, 54

carers vii, 9, 83-105

and engagement 94-8

guidance notes 114-16

involvement 58

mistaken beliefs 91

observable changes in the voice-hearer 85-90

strategies for 98-105

Chadwick, P. 57

client-centred approaches 51, 64-5

clinicians viii, 9, 49-82

guidance notes 113-14

orientation and attitude 57-61

outcome goals 53-7

therapeutic frameworks 64-81

ward staff training 51-2, 53

cognitive approaches 51, 65-73

cognitive behavioural approaches 51, 65-73

cognitive dissonance 66, 67-9, 82

Coleman, R. 72, 82

collaborative approach 51, 64-5

collusion 65

commands 54, 61, 68, 100

communication about voices 55, 59, 88, 101

compassionate mind approach 76-7

conditioning, operant 56, 82

confirmation bias 66, 82

conflict-causing behaviour 61

confusion 15, 20, 88

consistency, internal 59

constructive control vii

Ⓡ Routledge
Taylor & Francis Group

contact, maintaining 59

content targets 121

control 104

coping 10-12, 53-5, 99-102

criticism 24, 37, 38, 39

. . . .

déjà vu feelings 29

denial 87

desensitisation 18, 63, 70, 82

development 80

dialogue 36, 47, 55, 71-3, 82, 100-1

displacement activities 71, 82

distraction *see* avoidance strategies

distress 24, 89, 90

drugs

    medication 3, 6, 8, 56, 92, 123

    misuse of 29, 89, 92, 94

early intervention 58-9

emergencies flowchart 122

emotions 8

    experienced by carers and family 85-7

    misinterpreting normal experiences 28, 29

    spectrum of 13-14

    thoughts, actions and 12-20

emotions–thoughts–actions cycle 14-15, 19, 43

empowerment 121

engagement 78

    carers and family 94-8

Erikson, E. 80

Escher, S. 10, 52, 56, 69

events 14, 15-16

    emergencies flowchart 122

    good events and stress 26

    trauma and voices 43-4

existential proactive strategy 43-4

experiences

    anomalous 19, 20, 65

    misinterpreting normal experiences 26-30

    and personal meaning 4-6, 43-4, 103

. . . .

Fadden, G. 70-1

faking 59

family 83-105

    and engagement 94-8

    environment 75

    guidance notes 114-16

    involvement 58

    observable changes in the voice-hearer 87-90

    strategies for 98-105

fear 8, 16-17

feelings–thoughts–actions cycle 14-15, 19, 43

    see also emotions

Festinger, L. 67, 82

focusing 11, 19, 55, 63-4, 101-2

    vs avoidance 70-3

Frusciante, J. 23

. . . .

Garety, P. 57

gender of the voice 34

general system theory 74, 82

goals, clinician's 53-7

good voices 54, 99-100

GPs 76, 87

R Routledge
Taylor & Francis Group

grief 87

group effects 28

group therapy 69

group for voice-hearers 52-3

Hage, P. 10, 72, 123

Haley, J. 56, 60, 73

history of voice hearing 34, 59, 80-1, 82, 124-5

hostage situations 74

imploding 99

imposterism 7

'in spite of' strategy 40-1

ineffective strategies 45

information gathering 103-4

    process history 34, 59, 80-1, 82, 124-5

    voice profile 34-6, 126-7

intense thinking 29

internal consistency 59

interpersonal-relationship framework 73-4

interpretations 4-6, 15, 54, 103, 121

invitation strategy 42-3

isolation, social 60, 78, 89

Jayne, J. 123

Jeffers, S. 3

laughter 35

loss

    carers and family 85-7

    major personal loss 28

louder voices 62

lying to the voices 41

Maslow, A. vi-vii

McMillen, K. iv

meanings 4-6, 43-4, 103

medical approach 6

medication 3, 6, 8, 56, 92, 123

medico-legal risk assessment 61

memories 5-6, 29

mental capacity 60, 82

metaphor 60

mindfulness 77

misattribution 65

misinterpreting normal experiences 26-30

mistaken beliefs, carers' 91

Mittelmann, B. vi-vii

Morison, A. 57

mystery 7, 80

name, voice's 34

narrative approach 52, 80-1

negotiation 96-8

Nietzsche, F. iv, 15, 54, 103

normalising 42

normality vi-vii

    misinterpreting normal experiences 26-30

operant conditioning 56, 82

opinions 54, 100

organisation phase 12

orientation, clinician's 57-61

outcome goals, clinician's 53-7

panic 70

paradox 60, 82

Ｒ Routledge
Taylor & Francis Group

paradoxical intention 42-3

peer group 75

perception 54, 68

personal interpretations 4-6, 15, 54, 103, 121

personal responses 121

phases of hearing voices 12, 33

phobias 63

Piaget, J. 80

positive voices 54, 99-100

power 8, 9, 33, 51, 54

    carers/families and voices' power 98-9

    positions in a relationship 73-4

    sources of voices' power 25-30

pragmatism 93-4

predictability 96

proactive special tricks 40-6

problem of cause 3-4

problem-solving techniques 70-1

process history 34, 59, 80-1, 82, 124-5

process targets 121

progress assessment sheet 129

progression of change 92-3

psychiatry 3

psycho-social approach 3-4, 20

public, risks to the 61

recovery vii

reframing 66-7, 69

relapse prevention 58-9, 130

relapse signature 59, 130

relationships 9, 30

    changed between carer or family and voice hearer 93-4

interpersonal-relationship framework 73-4

request strategy 41-3

resilience factors vii, 20

risk assessment 60-1

risk taking 60

Romme, M. 52, 56, 69, 72, 123

    coping 10-12, 53-5, 99-101

    phases of hearing voices 12, 33

    progression of change 92-3

Sainsbury Centre for Mental Health 95

Sarason, I.G. 85-6

seeing voices in a different light 11, 54, 99-100

selective listening 39-40

self-defeating processes/behaviour 57, 65, 82

self-harm 15, 60-1, 89, 92, 101

self-knowledge 96

self-respect 36, 39

self-worth 15, 20, 36-40, 76, 80, 119

set-ups 79, 82

sleep deprivation 28

social contact 78

social isolation 60, 78, 89

Solly, A. 77

specialist medical unit 76

spectrum of feelings 13-14

stabilisation phase 12

startling phase 12, 33, 89

statements/opinions 54, 100

strategies 128

    for carers and families 98-105

    strategic overview 121

    for voice-hearers 40-6

stress 25-6

subordinate role 73-4

substance abuse 15, 29, 89, 92, 94

suicide attempts 60-1, 76

Sun Tzu 70

symptoms 85-9

systems approach 74-6, 82

....

therapeutic techniques 56-7, 64-81

  awareness of set-ups 79

  behavioural 65-73

  breaking the isolation 78

  client-centred 51, 64-5

  cognitive 51, 65-73

  cognitive behavioural 51, 65-73

  collaborative 51, 64-5

  compassionate mind 76-7

  interpersonal-relationship 73-4

  mindfulness 77

  narrative 52, 80-1

  pursuing a valued role 78

  systems approach 74-6, 82

thoughts 29

  automatic negative thoughts 28, 29

  emotions, actions and 12-20

  feelings–thoughts–actions cycle 14-15, 19, 43

tranquillisers 8

trauma 28-9, 43-4, 81

trouble-causing behaviour 61

trust 95

....

universality 69

....

valued role 78

voice-hearers vii, 9, 21-47

  changing the way of thinking about voices 30-3

  guidance notes 110-13

  paying attention to self-worth 36-40

  proactive special tricks 40-6

  sources of voices' power 25-30

  symptoms 85-9

voice profile 34-6, 126-7

voices 1-20

  bad and good 54, 99-100

  communication about 55, 59, 88, 101

  guidance notes 110

  information gathering about 34-6, 126-7

  nature of 23-5

  problem of cause 3-4

  seeing them in a different light 11, 54, 99-100

  understanding 6-20

  weak 23

Von Bertalanffy, L. 76

vulnerabilities 96

Vygotsky, L.S. 80

....

ward staff training 51-2, 53

Watzlawick, P. 66, 72

weak voices 23

withdrawal 60, 78, 89

Yalom, I.D. 52, 57, 69